Claiming Power over Life

Hastings Center Studies in Ethics

A SERIES EDITED BY

Gregory E. Kaebnick and Daniel Callahan

Established in 1969, The Hastings Center, located in Garrison, New York, is an independent, nonprofit, and nonpartisan research organization that examines ethical issues in medicine and the life sciences. The work of the Center is mainly carried out through research projects, the publication of the *Hastings Center Report* and *IRB: A Review of Human Subjects Research*, and numerous workshops, conferences, lectures, and consultations. The *Hastings Center Studies in Ethics* is a series intended to bring the ongoing research work of The Hastings Center to a wider audience.

Claiming Power over Life
Religion and Biotechnology Policy

Mark J. Hanson, Editor

GEORGETOWN UNIVERSITY PRESS / WASHINGTON, D.C.

Georgetown University Press, Washington, D.C. 20007
© 2001 by Georgetown University Press. All rights reserved.
Printed in the United States of America
10   9   8   7   6   5   4   3   2   1   2001
THIS VOLUME IS PRINTED ON ACID-FREE OFFSET BOOK PAPER

Library of Congress Cataloging-in-Publication Data

Claiming power over life : religion and biotechnology policy / Mark J. Hanson,
    editor.
        p. cm. — (Hastings Center studies in ethics)
    Includes index.
    ISBN 0-87840-864-9 (alk. paper)
    1. Biotechnology—Religious aspects. 2. Medical technology—Religious
aspects. I. Hanson Mark J. II. Series.
TP248.23 .C535 2001
291.1'75—dc21   2001023261

CONTENTS

Acknowledgments

This book is the outcome of a three-year research project titled "Religion and Biotechnology Project," organized by The Hastings Center and part of a larger "Values and Biotechnology" initiative. Projects in this initiative were funded in part by grants from the H. Goldsmith Foundation, the Monsanto Company, and The Hastings Center.

I would like to thank the many project participants who participated in rich discussions on project issues and who thereby helped advance the work of the project as well as, I am sure, the thinking of the authors in this volume: Judith Andre (Michigan State University), Gary Barton (Monsanto Company), Baruch Brody (Baylor College of Medicine), Lisa Sowle Cahill (Boston College), Courtney Campbell (Oregon State University), Audrey Chapman (American Association for the Advancement of Science), James J. Childress (University of Virginia), Ronald Cole-Turner (Pittsburgh Theological Seminary), Robert Collier (Monsanto Company), Gary Comstock (Iowa State University), Harold Edgar (Columbia Law School), John Evans (University of Southern California, Los Angeles), Margaret Farley (Yale Divinity School), Mark Frankel (American Association of the Advancement of Science), E. Richard Gold (University of Western Ontario), Vigen Guroian (Loyola College, Baltimore), Jaydee Hanson (United Methodist Board of Church and Society), Cathleen Kaveny (Notre Dame Law School), Gail Kempler (Regeneron Pharmaceuticals, Inc.), B. Andrew Lustig (Rice University), Gerald McKenny (University of Notre Dame), Gilbert Milaender (Valparaiso University), C. Ben Mitchell (The Southern Baptist Theological Seminary), Jill Montgomery (Monsanto Company), Dorothy Nelkin (New York University), Sara Radcliffe (SmithKline Beecham Pharmaceuticals), Larry Rassmussen (Union Theological Seminary), Leslie S. Rothenberg (University of California, Los Angeles), Abdulaziz Sachedina (University of Virginia), David Schmickel (Biotechnology Industry Organization), Roger Shinn (Union Theological Seminary), Frank Stokes (Monsanto Company), Suzanne Tomlinson (Biotechnology Industry Organization), Virginia Weldon (Monsanto Company), Gillian Woollett

(Pharmaceutical Research and Manufacturers of America), and Michael Yesley (Los Alamos National Laboratory).

I would also like to thank the staff of The Hastings Center at that time, with special thanks to Leigh Turner, research associate; Nicole Rozanski, administrative assistant; and the staff of the *Hastings Center Report*, Bette-Jane Crigger, Erika Blacksher, Amy Menasché, and Mary-Anne Dahlia.

The chapter "Religious Voices in Biotechnology: The Case of Gene Patenting" originally appeared as a special supplement in the *Hastings Center Report* 27, no. 6 (1997): S1–S21.

John H. Evans's chapter, "The Uneven Playing Field of the Dialogue of Patenting," is a revised version of an essay that was published in Audrey R. Chapman, ed., *Perspectives on Genetic Patenting: Religion, Science and Industry in Dialogue* (Washington, D.C.: American Association for the Advancement of Science, 1999), pp. 57–73. It is being used with the permission of the Program of Dialogue on Science, Ethics, and Religion of the American Association for the Advancement of Science.

Audrey R. Chapman's chapter is based on *Unprecedented Choices: Religious Ethics at the Frontiers of Genetic Science* by Audrey R. Chapman, copyright © 1999 Augsburg Fortress (ISBN 0-8006-3181-1). Reprinted by permission.

Elliot N. Dorff's chapter has been slightly revised and is excerpted from a longer entry, "Religious Views on Biotechnology: Jewish," in the *Encyclopedia of Ethical, Legal, and Policy Issues in Biotechnology*, ed. Thomas H. Murray and Maxwell Mehleman, pp. 924–38, copyright © 2000 by John Wiley & Sons, Inc. Reprinted by permission of John Wiley & Sons, Inc.

MARK J. HANSON

Introduction

Rapid advances in biotechnology are prompting many people to raise questions and make statements about it that sound distinctively religious. The human genome is described publicly as the "book of life" and the "holy grail." In his announcement of the completion of the map of the human genome, director of the National Human Genome Research Institute, Francis Collins, called the genome "our own instruction book, previously known only to God." This kind of religious language symbolizes the kind of power that human beings, through biotechnology, are obtaining over the biological components of life itself. Whatever it means to play God, we surely seem to be closer to it than ever before.

It is not surprising, therefore, that religious traditions are taking an increasing interest in biotechnology. To be sure, their attention to issues raised by biomedical technology generally is not new. But novel technologies are generating questions and choices that humanity has not had to face before. The answers to these questions and justifiability of many choices prompted by biotechnology rely on assumptions regarding the meaning of human life, the limits of our ambitions to eliminate contingency and enhance ourselves and nature, the extent of our powers over reproduction, the nature of the relationships between human and nonhuman life, the proper level of control over mechanisms of life and death, and so on.

These are the sorts of issues on which religious traditions should have something to say. These traditions are bearers of the centuries of human wisdom and have shaped the values and behaviors of human cultures through the ages. Can they now provide insight and guidance not only to their followers but also to the broader public moral discourse and policy debates that will establish public policy around such difficult questions?

The theological and philosophical depths of the issues raised by biotechnology are also providing significant challenges to the assumptions that normally inform policymaking in the United States. Policymaking in liberal democracies is guided by the central notion that policies should not be justified in the terms of any particular tradition's understanding of what constitutes a good human life. Public policy debates often then reduce to the central concerns of liberalism, namely maximizing individual freedoms and minimizing tangible harms. The complexity of issues raised by biotechnology is testing the adequacy of relying on these assumptions in public discourse and policymaking. A more direct engagement with richer religious and philosophical traditions may be necessary for a more adequate debate.

A Hastings Center project studied the intersection of religion and biotechnology policy in relation to two developments that made headlines and elicited responses from policymakers and religious leaders alike. In 1995, nearly 200 religious leaders signed an appeal against human and animal patenting. And in 1996, the first successful somatic cell nuclear transfer cloning technique to produce a live animal—the famous sheep, Dolly—prompted widespread public policy discussions with substantial input from religious thinkers and leaders. What subsequent dialogues among religious leaders, policymakers, and the biotechnology industry made clear was that religious traditions had much work to do to be able to interpret these new developments within their own traditions of wisdom, and that policy discourse was impoverished by an inability to accommodate religious insights in productive ways. Theological and ethical development, as well as maturation of ways of reasoning in the public square, are needed to address adequately the emerging challenges of biotechnology.

The chapters in this volume address these themes in varying ways. They advance our thinking on these matters, and point to new directions for further work.

In his chapter, "Meaningful Resistance: Religion and Biotechnology," Courtney Campbell reminds readers that religion is not a newcomer to public discourse about biotechnology and biomedicine. Current controversies, however, have prompted procedural and substantive objections to the value of religious discourse and perspectives in public policy. Campbell examines prospects for constructive contributions from religion. He begins by offering a model of religious communities in democratic societies he calls "meaningful resistance," a contrast to a model of exclusion presupposed in liberal political theory and bioethics. Religions acknowledge their own authorities while attesting to the issues of meaning that are opened up by biotechnology. Then, using the debates surrounding gene patenting and cloning as context, he provides an assessment of arguments opposing religion in public discourse. Campbell's conclusion is that there are methods by which "religions of resistance can nonetheless infuse meaning into social disputes over the ethics of biotechnology."

B. Andrew Lustig, in "Human Cloning and Liberal Neutrality: Why We Need to Broaden the Public Dialogue," considers possibilities of drawing parallels between religious and nonreligious arguments. He argues that while religious arguments are distinctive, their character is "functionally equivalent" to certain nonreligious arguments. In the context of the debate on human cloning, Lustig observes a kind of "common ground" between religious and nonreligious appeals that is suggestive of a notion of the "common good." He argues that certain themes in communitarian thought can offer correctives to the narrow assumptions of recent political theory, and concludes by considering how a wider understanding of public reasoning can more readily incorporate appeals to broader aesthetic, moral, or religiously based concerns.

My chapter, "Religious Voices in Biotechnology: The Case of Gene Patenting," is a synthetic analysis of the research and project meetings of The Hastings Center's project activities related to the gene patenting debate beginning in 1995. It describes the debate primarily in terms of an intersection of three realms of values: the legal system, the biotechnology industry, and religion. I argue that failure to attend to the values dimensions of the debate in appropriate ways led to miscommunication among representatives of these realms and charges that religious leaders were merely ignorant of genetic science and the patent system. I make recommendations for future dialogue, both on the patenting issues specifically and for issues at the intersection of religion and biotechnology generally. I found that study of the patenting controversy serves as an excellent case study for this latter set of issues.

In "The Uneven Playing Field of the Dialogue on Patenting," John Evans brings a sociological perspective to the intersection of religion and biotechnology. He uses the tool of looking at the issue and argumentative "frames" used by participants from the biotechnology industry and religious traditions in dialogues about patenting and finds that the "playing field" of dialogue is slanted against religious traditions. The issue has been framed as being about patenting itself, rather than the broader issue of the commodification of life, and arguments are framed in terms of ethical discourse, rather than prophetic discourse, to borrow James Gustafson's categories.[1] This latter framing owes to the bias toward ethical reasoning in policy decision making, emphasizing cost-benefit analysis and having little room for nuance and complexity in argument.

This has resulted in the "burden of proof" being on those employing prophetic language to "translate" their discourse into other terms, thereby losing effectiveness. Evans advocates for recognizing how these frames are used, a moratorium on insisting that opponents' arguments make sense in the others' frames, an insistence on the legitimacy of prophetic claims in the public realm (although not religious warrants for policy), and ultimately, the assertion of democracy in public debate involving a wider selection of citizens, rather than allowing debates to be shaped merely by the "elite." Neglecting prophetic claims will leave significant issues unattended.

In "Religious Perspectives on Biotechnology," Audrey R. Chapman provides a comprehensive review of the religious perspectives on biotechnology over the last twenty years and recognizes their contributions as well as their shortcomings. She believes that their success has been in sensitizing and stimulating the moral imagination of religious and secular publics, identifying values and commitments challenged by genetics, expanding ethical horizons, and making clear that "nothing less is at stake than the moral compass and fundamental humanity of ours and future societies." Nonetheless, they have done more to raise questions than provide answers. Like Evans, she recognizes the difficulties of using a prophetic form of discourse in public debates but argues that religious traditions could employ the form with more effective reasoning than has been the case. Chapman also outlines how religious thinkers could use "public theology" more effectively. Given their emphasis on broader social values, such as justice and human dignity and the common good, religious traditions have much to offer the public debates about biotechnology. But Chapman believes that religious ethicists must do more to offer real normative guidance, given the unprecedented challenges that biotechnology brings.

Ronald Cole-Turner undertakes Chapman's challenge by beginning with the question, What can theology learn from genetics and biotechnology? Building on modest beginnings within academic theology, Cole-Turner makes progress on this question by looking at classic themes of Christian theology—God the creator, creation, freedom and moral responsibility, and humans in relation to nature—rather than specific technologies. For Cole-Turner, genetic science challenges us to reconsider how God creates, the extent of God's exercise of power, and God's relation to animals. We must also reconsider ourselves to be part of a dynamic and emergent process of evolutionary creation, as a nondualistic self, with a soul and a will defined in terms of capacities defined and constrained by biological and genetic factors. In light of the new powers granted us by the tools of biotechnology, we must also reconsider our roles within creation in relation to God's purposes.

Also advancing substantive theological considerations in relation to biotechnology is Gerald P. McKenny, with his chapter, "Religion, Biotechnology, and the Integrity of Nature: A Critical Examination." McKenny examines a fairly common but ill-defined theme that biotechnology violates in some way the "integrity of nature" or "life itself" and whether there are grounds in religious convictions for appropriate conflict between religious communities and the biotechnology industry. Roman Catholic statements deny a privileged role to DNA in characterizing human nature and identity, emphasizing normative concepts of nature and the natural order. Promoting the natural is given higher valuation than intervening with the artificial, such as with tools of biotechnology. Protestant and ecumenical documents, in contrast, emphasize the value of life itself and the central role of DNA in the essence of life. Genetic interventions involve a reductionism of life, ignoring its sacred quality, and therefore, when utilized on human beings, involve at least some violation of the sacredness or dignity of human life, even if that intervention may be justifiable by its benefits. McKenny concludes that conflicts between religious traditions and biotechnology on the basis of these themes will ultimately be rare. He suggests how biotechnology redescribes nature and life, and articulates central challenges for Christianity to provide critiques of the aims, desires, and norms of biotechnology in light of the commitments of Christian ethics, and to affirm, "against the incremental utopianism of much of the biotechnology industry, the intractable otherness of nature that on this side of the resurrection resists the totalizing union with human aims, desires, and norms."

In "Jewish Views on Technology in Health Care," Elliot N. Dorff describes the foundations for Judaism's "activist, and yet respectful, stance toward the world and toward life and health" and then examines a variety of biomedical technologies applied to the beginning of life. Methodologically, Judaism uses Jewish law and theology together to give moral guidance. The Jewish orientation toward technology is that it is neither good nor bad in itself. Human beings were created and are therefore obligated "to bend God's world to God's purposes and ours—as long . . . as we preserve God's world in the process." Technology applied to health care should, according to Dorff, be applied by three principles: (1) God's ownership of our bodies; (2) the body as morally neutral and potentially good; and (3) human obligation to help other people escape sickness, injury, and death. Dorff then reviews Judaism's tradition of reasoning in the context of several biomedical technologies. Biotechnology, he argues, should be researched because of its potential benefits, but also applied cautiously, recognizing its moral and theological implications.

These essays provide a new agenda for meeting the challenges for various traditions to find ways to reason together in a more effective public discourse. The ethical and social implications of biotechnology are too important for these challenges not to be undertaken urgently.

NOTE

1. James M. Gustafson, "Moral Discourse about Medicine: A Variety of Forms," *The Journal of Medicine and Philosophy* 15 (1990): 125–42.

COURTNEY CAMPBELL

Meaningful Resistance: Religion and Biotechnology

Recent controversies about gene patenting and cloning have prompted renewed interest in understanding and analyzing the stake of religious communities in the biotechnological revolution. Yet, it is important to remember that the major faith traditions have played an important role in public discourse about biotechnology and biomedicine for a long period of time preceding the contemporary disputes. In the late 1970s, for example, as scientists began to initiate research on genetically engineered organisms, a letter was submitted to President Jimmy Carter by the leaders of national ecclesiastical bodies representing Judaism, Protestantism, and Roman Catholicism. The letter expressed concern about important values, such as human dignity, that might be challenged by genetic engineering, especially in the absence of public oversight and monitoring. President Carter directed a federal commission to examine these questions and evaluate the legitimacy of the concerns raised by the religious communities.[1]

A couple of important lessons can be gleaned from this episode. First, although vigorous criticism has been directed against giving a hearing to religious perspectives in current controversies in biotechnology or, particularly in the context of disputes over cloning, purportedly according public legitimization to certain (especially conservative) religious views,[2] it cannot be said that consideration of religious views is without precedent. Indeed, it can be argued that attention has been given to religious ideas and frameworks of reasoning in *every* national bioethics commission, beginning in the 1970s with the National Commission for the Protection of Human Subjects in Biomedical and Behavioral Research.[3] Second, the ecumenical letter addressing genetic engineering offers an important model of religious involvement in public policy for both advocates and critics, in which religious communities *unite*, not with common answers and policy solutions, but with *questions* they wish to ensure are not neglected by deliberative bodies, as well as the scientific community and the biotechnological industry.

Nonetheless, the current controversies in biotechnology have prompted both procedural and substantive objections to the value of religious discourse and perspectives in public policy. Some of these objections have the practical implication of disqualifying religious voices and traditions from receiving serious and fair consideration within the moral and political communities. At issue here is not only the cogency of arguments and positions advanced from a religious tradition, but more generally, competing visions about the public space that can legitimately be claimed by a religious community.

In this chapter, I want to examine the prospects for constructive contributions from traditions of religious thought in the context of new developments in biotechnology and biomedicine. I will begin by sketching a model of religious community in a democratic society that I will refer to as "meaningful resistance." This account presents striking contrasts with the model of exclusion of religion presupposed in liberal political theory and expressed in bioethics critiques. I will then turn to an overview of the specific philosophical and political critiques directed at religious perspectives on biotechnology, particularly within the context of debates over gene patenting and cloning, and assess the validity of these arguments. I will conclude the essay by suggesting methods by which religions of resistance can nonetheless infuse meaning into social disputes over the ethics of biotechnology.

Religious Community: Authority and Influence

In beginning, it is worth asking why it is that public policy bodies have repeatedly addressed the views of religious traditions in debates over bioethics. What is it that the values and positions of such traditions have to offer for commissions authorized to reflect on new controversies precipitated by advances in biotechnology and to make recommendations about social funding and directions for scientific research? James F. Childress, a leading proponent of inclusionary public policy in bioethics, has suggested several possibilities.[4] Childress contends that a responsible public policy must attend to the issues of concern for all citizens and seek to ensure that policy conclusions can be defended and justified before a broad audience of citizens, including members of religious communities. Strong support or opposition from religious communities can provide an important marker for the political feasibility of a policy recommendation. In addition, religious communities constitute historical traditions of moral wisdom, and thus provide "ethical background" for understanding and interpreting an embedded social morality. Indeed, in certain respects, Childress is willing to maintain that what is termed "secularization," is not, as often claimed, the separation of society from religion, but rather involves the institutionalization of historical religious norms in social practices.[5]

This case for inclusion is more procedural than substantive, in that religious warrants are held to be no longer required for basic norms such as liberty, mutual respect, equality, and fairness, even though such warrants can provide historical and motivational backing for adhering to such values in the formation of public policy. Social commitments to fair procedures and equal opportunity require a hearing for the perspectives articulated by religious traditions, no less so than those formulated by philosophic, medical, or scientific traditions. Moreover, the substantive claims of religious traditions can shape and illuminate the "overlapping consensus" of society's core morality.[6] In short, religious traditions can be integral to the policy process, even if not specifically invoked as a warrant for a policy recommendation.

A second inclusionary rationale is that religious traditions often raise "objections" that are important to identify and evaluate in the presence of strong scientific, industry, and political pressures to pursue a line of biotechnological research. In the context of biomedical policy, where prospective outcomes and consequences of research carry tremendous weight but are difficult to assess accurately, religious "objections" may be particularly important to consider because they commonly rely on matters of intrinsic value that cannot be reduced to a circumstantialist ethic. This rationale directs attention more to the substance of religious concerns than to due process, but evaluating the normative legitimacy of substantive religious issues can itself be a daunting task for a policy body. In addition, a focus on religious "objections" may unfairly cast faith traditions always in the role of "naysayer" and an "obstacle to progress" in scientific research or to biotechnology in the view of the public as a whole, even as religious "support" for certain practices is neglected. Nonetheless, as illustrated by my initial example of the concerns raised by religious traditions about gene splicing, these "objections" can elicit sustained examination of practices or questions that might otherwise be overlooked.

Whether the argument for inclusion of religious views is procedural or substantive, it is not compelling to many critics, who may advocate a policy process that is exclusionary and immune from religious influence. Indeed, supporters of an exclusionary position may assess policy contexts that take religious thought seriously to be "odd" and even reflective of a "bias" in favor of religion.[7] Such positions are ultimately rooted in an interpretation of liberal political theory that affirms strict separation of the religious from the political realm. On this view, the parameters of civic discourse in a democratic society preclude consideration of explicit religious claims, values, and positions. While such values are important as action guides and sources of meaning within the religious community, they should carry no weight in public discourse.

I want to offer a contrasting model of religious community in a democratic society that draws on the arguments advanced by law professor Stephen L. Carter concerning an "ideal of religious autonomy."[8] Carter in turn is indebted to the insights of Alexis de Tocqueville about the interrelationships of religious belief and the values of freedom and equality, and the significance of civil associations, such as religious communities, as intermediate communities between the self and state. Of critical importance in de Tocqueville's observations is a distinction between *authority* and *influence*. De Tocqueville is quite convinced that the religious communities of the new American republic are influential precisely because they have forsworn political authority and power.[9] Having given up theocratic aspirations and establishmentarian relations with the federal government, religiosity flourishes to a degree that de Tocqueville finds astonishing and instructive for his continental peers. Indeed, a play for political power by a religious association will undercut the very vitality of the religion: "Any alliance with any political power whatsoever is bound to be burdensome for religion. It does not need their support in order to live, and in serving them it may die."[10]

Relying on this distinction, permitting and even inviting religious discourse in public policy can be understood as an acknowledgment and expression of the *influence* of religion, but does not constitute a ceding of *authority* (moral, political, etc.) to religion. Such discourse should be considered neither odd, nor reflective of political bias, but instead compatible with both the principles of freedom of expression and of separation of church and state. The separationist principle (which de Tocqueville clearly endorses) primarily concerns itself with issues of authority and authorization in society, as manifested through law and policy. Religious discourse may have influence on the *process* of formulating law and policy, but the authorization or *warrant* for a specific law ultimately rests (or should rest) on nonreligious grounds.

The contemporary interest and even insistence of public policy commissions in eliciting the "objections" of religious traditions is an important illustration of this distinction. The "objections" to human cloning, to gene patenting, to genetic analysis of human tissue samples, to neocortical brain death, and so on, claim influence on religious adherents. Insofar as these adherents are also citizens, such claims hold influence for other citizens in the role of policymakers. The influence of religious objections may also be displayed when certain restraints on otherwise permissible conduct are respected and institutionalized, such as exemptions to a medical procedure based on religious claims (e.g., objection to autopsy). These objections do not, however, have the authoritative status or enforceability of law for the citizenry taken as a whole. De Tocqueville's distinction, when applied to the current interplay of scientific freedom, the ethics of biotechnology, and religious questions, seems almost prescient: "While the law allows the American people to do everything, there are things which religion prevents them from imagining and forbids them to dare."[11]

Carter's account of the autonomy of religions borrows and extends the insights of de Tocqueville. The expression of religious ideas in public discourse constitutes neither an "establishment" nor an "imposition" of religion. That language presumes categories of political power and authority, not influence through freedom of expression. Indeed, Carter's interpretation of religious community requires a strong wall of separation between religious and political authority. This enables religions to serve two primary functions in a democratic society: "First, they can serve as the sources of moral understanding without which any majoritarian system can deteriorate into simple tyranny, and second, they can mediate between the citizen and the apparatus of government, providing an independent moral voice."[12] This is a very different model of religious community than the private, sealed enclaves presupposed in liberal political theory, and some exposition of this position is necessary.

It is significant that one common thread in Carter's interpretation is the ethical insight embedded in religious communities. The principal characteristic of moral understanding Carter attributes to religions is "the power of resistance," or the courage and integrity to affirm certain moral values as ultimate in such a way that they deny *authority* to the dominant social institutions, including political institutions.[13] In a democratic society, resistance is an essential feature of religion. Thus, it should not be surprising that religious traditions do have "objections" to aspects of contemporary life, including developments in biotechnology. Such objections are a sign of a flourishing and vibrant religion, whereas the absence of objection, the absence of resistance, or accommodation once the scientific issues have been resolved, is a mark of a deformed and even deadened religious conscience.

The possibility of religious objection and resistance resides, however, in the "autonomy of religions," that is, that religions possess an "independence" from dominant social institutions, especially the state (but also from science or the corporate world). Like de Tocqueville, Carter's claim is that religious influence is conditioned by the degree of distance erected and maintained between the religious and political realm. This moral independence enables the religious community to affirm fidelity to its fundamental value commitments in two important ways. First, a community must be autonomous for its resistance to patterns and practices in the broader society to be authentic and credible. Second, this autonomy provides social space for the religious community to conduct its internal ecclesiastical affairs (e.g., spousal relationships, sexual ethics, women as priests) according to its own value commitments and independent of intrusion by other social institutions. This enables religious communities to embody "alternative sources of meaning for their adherents,"[14] a particularly vital function when, as some commentators have observed, bioethics must deliberately neglect questions of meaning in order to pursue consensus.[15]

The contrasts between Carter's political ecclesiology and the views of liberal political theorists who have been influential in demarcating the social context of bioethics are important to delineate. First, Carter portrays his understanding of religious community as simultaneously "subversive" and necessary to democracy. Carter's model enables religious traditions to offer forms of prophetic criticism against society and biomedical science, criticisms that may be influential for adherents, policymakers, or professional bodies, but also involves a renunciation of aspirations to authority and dominance in the political realm. This is quite different than theoretical approaches that seek to render religion politically invisible and/or ethically dispensable in democratic society, and which find themselves continually suspicious of religious imperialism and of theocratic pretensions.

Second, liberal political theorists, beginning with Hobbes and Locke, have made the principal (and for some, the only) moral and political question to turn on the relationship between the self and the state. The self is thereby extracted from his or her community and life context. Carter's political ecclesiology, by contrast, embeds the self within various mediating communities, including family and religious community, which issues in a diverse (and different) set of *primary* moral relations and obligations. It is through these mediating relations, moreover, that access is opened to personal and collective sources of meaning and purpose, toward which the liberal state has declared itself to be agnostic.

Third, many religious commentators in bioethics have expressed dismay over the preeminence accorded to the principle of respect for autonomy or self-determination in bioethical decision making. The sovereignty of autonomy seems not only to encompass personal choices, such as reproductive rights or termination of life, but also is presumed in policy contexts. Thus, in the policy debate over human cloning, arguments against proceeding with cloning had to overcome a moral and political presumption in favor of the freedom of scientific inquiry and reproductive autonomy. The implication of Carter's view, however, is that autonomy is not as antithetical to religious thought as has commonly been suggested. Indeed, freedom from state intrusiveness is absolutely vital to authentic religious expression and resistance. Substantive religious claims in bioethics thereby presuppose procedural guarantees of the autonomy of religions. Such autonomy gives religious communities and religious thought a legitimate social space within the democratic state.

My claim is that critiques of religious thought in the context of the ethics of biotechnology conflate the distinction between influence and authority, such that expression of religious perspectives in public discourse is interpreted as an "imposition" of religion, a veiled grab for political authority. This interpretation of religion in a context of power leads to misguided calls for marginalization or exclusion of religious discourse from spheres of bioethics policymaking. I want to provide a closer, and critical, examination of these critiques, particularly as they emerged in the dispute over human cloning in the late 1990s.

Religion as Subversive Authority

Certainly, religious discourse and religious communities no longer are held in the high social esteem that de Tocqueville commented upon in the mid-nineteenth century. Within philosophical bioethics, religious traditions are often seen less as a repository of moral wisdom and more as an anachronistic residue of pre-Enlightenment social organization, which should have minimal bearing on contemporary debates in the liberal democratic state. As illustrated in the writings of Rawls and in contemporary commentators in bioethics, a cohesive and coherent social morality requires the public invisibility of religion. The public door on religious thought, it is argued, needs to remain firmly in place, lest society risks rekindling the animosity and violence of the wars of religion or their contemporary discursive counterpart, the "culture wars."[16]

These critiques presume certain characteristics to religious discourse and community that require further exposition in order to assess their validity. For the critique ultimately aims to construct a "religion-free" zone for public policy. Religious communities and traditions, by contrast, constitute subversive authorities characterized by absolutism, authoritarianism, fatalism, and divisiveness.

Absolutism

Part of the appeal of including religious perspectives in the policy process, as noted above, is that these positions many times are stated in "absolute" terms because they are rooted in intrinsic values at the core of a tradition's moral identity. Instead of piling qualification upon qualification in a manner approximate to the complex circumstances that must be addressed by legal, political, and some philosophical positions (such as casuistry), some religious traditions may affirm flat prohibitions on certain scientific practices or biotechnological applications. In this respect, absolutism has the advantage of clarity, while potentially lacking specificity and comprehensiveness.

However, as the policy focus shifts from process to outcome, and there is pressure—corporate, legal, political, scientific, philosophical, or otherwise—to come to consensus on both the values that are shared and/or the practices that are recommended,[17] absolutes can prove very resistant to incorporation. The web of policymaking in democratic life is permeated by negotiation and compromise, but it is the nature of an absolute to be nonnegotiable.[18] Thus, insofar as religious views on biotechnology are informed by certain absolute values (e.g., the claim of children to be born through sexual intercourse to genetically related parents), they can present seemingly insurmountable obstacles to consensus. Moreover, following a line of criticism popularized by Joseph Fletcher, a reliance on the absolutes embedded in Western religious morality seems to get the moral situation backwards, as principles take priority over persons.[19] It thus is not uncommon to hear complaints that a religious argument that seeks to limit or prohibit a biotechnological application is callous or insensitive to suffering, such as the suffering experienced by an infertile couple.

In commenting critically on the undue legitimization of religious perspectives by the National Bioethics Advisory Commission (NBAC) in its report on human cloning, Harvard biologist R. C. Lewontin alludes to another problem with absolutist religious arguments: "The immense strength of a religious viewpoint is that it is capable of abolishing hard ethical problems if only we can correctly decipher the meaning of what has been revealed to us. . . . The painful tensions and contradictions [on cloning] . . . that demand de facto resolution in public and private action did not appear in the testimony of any of the theologians [testifying before NBAC]."[20] While Lewontin's empirical observations are astonishingly superficial and mistaken, his theoretical point is certainly compelling: An absolutist position eliminates moral dilemmas. This is as true of Kant's categorical imperative or Mill's utilitarian principle as it is of a religious judgment rooted in the sanctity of human life. Thus, while *any* absolutist position will dissolve moral dilemmas in favor of the supreme or primary ethical principle, a position need not be *religious* to be absolutist.

What really makes religious argumentation on cloning (or gene patenting) problematic is not that it abolishes the moral dilemma, but rather that it *creates* one. The primary rationale advanced in favor of permitting cloning stems, as noted above, from what has become the moral trump in contemporary culture and bioethics, the principle of respect for autonomy. That is, autonomy, whether to defend freedom of scientific inquiry or to justify (more) reproductive choices, has itself been elevated to the status of an absolute. Its primacy is suggested by philosopher Gregory Pence, who contends that autonomy places choices about cloning humans beyond moral scrutiny and criticism.[21] When the cloning of human beings is described as "rais[ing] no moral issue" on grounds of autonomous choice over reproduction, then clearly what is at work is a moral absolute that has eliminated the "hard ethical problems." Religious values then must create whatever *moral* dilemmas are embedded in human cloning because philosophical bioethics offers no counterbalance to autonomy.

Carter's account requires us, however, to examine more closely the relation of religious absolutes and the principle of respect for autonomy. The vitality of a religious tradition in a democratic society presumes respect for the autonomy of religions. In that respect, autonomy is an absolute principle of *procedural morality* even for religious communities. Second, religious absolutes (and even religious nonabsolutes) create rather than dissolve moral dilemmas when "choice" and respect for autonomy are defended as an absolute principle of *substantive morality*. It is important to affirm the distinction between a procedural right to choose and a substantive right choice; religious argumentation has been very skeptical of letting the latter be defined only by an appeal to the former.

It also is the case that, in the dispute over human cloning, the critique of religious absolutism is misguided with respect to many specific faith communities. There are certainly some traditions that have declared a resolute "no" to human cloning, but even these traditions may differ with respect to the morality of animal, embryo, or plant cloning, and other aspects of the biotechnological revolution. Still other religious traditions have adopted what has been designated an "amberlight" position with respect to all of the above practices,[22] meaning they advocate caution, a slow approach to cloning and biotechnology, a careful assessment of the risks and benefits in proceeding, and erring on the side of safety. Thus, there are sound reasons for suspicion of the rejection of religious arguments on the grounds of their inflexible absolutism.

Authoritarian

Given secular culture's emphasis on autonomy, it is not surprising that religious views critical of a purely procedural morality of self-determination are often considered authoritarian. Religious argumentation that raises important questions about biotechnology may be described as "imposing" the moral authority of a religious tradition on personal, communal, or industry choices, and hence dismissed on grounds of dogmatism. That is, the claims are held to rely on convictions embedded in some of the foundational tenets or narratives of a religious tradition. These sources are somewhat obscure or inaccessible to the ordinary citizen and thus the claims embedded in them are seemingly immune from critical examination and refutation.

In the cases of both gene patenting and human cloning, the accusation of authoritarianism is repeatedly raised when religious scholars or commentators appeal to scripture, particularly the Genesis creation accounts, in the arguments. When these narratives are invoked to describe patterns of reasoning or to explicate the meaning of concepts internal to a tradition, such as the image of God, then the accusation is not valid. However, if the narratives or concepts are used to *prescribe* a normative point or claim, then the authoritarian objection must be looked at more carefully. In the first instance, a normative claim derived from a biblical narrative prompts important hermeneutical issues about why a given passage or story carries moral weight. That is, questions can be asked about the basis for its relevance to the question at hand, and the method of interpretation and application to the specific biotechnological issue.[23] If the normative claim is extended as a warrant for the adoption of a specific policy, then the concerns about theological imperialism and "imposing religion" gain greater credibility.

Here again, though, de Tocqueville's distinction between religious influence and political authority is compelling. A religious claim about biotechnology may gain influence in public discourse not because of its narrative source, but because it resonates with values that members of the society have accepted on other nonreligious grounds. This is entirely compatible with the moral logic of persuasion in a pluralistic society. By contrast, citizens are unlikely to find persuasive an appeal merely to biblical authority or the authority of tradition. Moreover, to mandate such a view for society solely on the basis of biblical authority would fall under the logic of coercion, because citizens would be unable to consent to such a position, and even their assent would not be informed. It is nonetheless the case that an *idea* central to religious traditions, such as the protection of the vulnerable and powerless in society (e.g., children in the case of human cloning), may have influence even if its originating *source* is not accepted as authoritative by the society.

The hermeneutical and interpretative issues embedded in appeals to scriptural warrants were strikingly on display in religious testimony on human cloning before NBAC. For example, both Jewish rabbis and Christian theologians invoked the creation account in Genesis as a hermeneutical starting point for understanding human nature, but *different* passages were cited to lend support for quite different conclusions. Jewish rabbis invoked Genesis 2, which presents a delegation of "dominion" to human beings. In Jewish thought, this delegation of responsibility is understood to imply that creation is incomplete and broken, and humans are under an imperative to mend and heal creation. Thus, Jewish thinkers could envision rare circumstances, such as last-resort measures to preserve genealogical lineage or to overcome infertility, under which cloning would be consistent with the responsibility of dominion.

Christian theologians, meanwhile, often cited Genesis 1, wherein human beings are revealed as created in the divine image (*imago Dei*). This provided a basis for a normative critique of cloning and other biotechnological procedures that enable creation of others after our own image (*imago mei*). While not conclusive, the moral weight attributed to this passage helps explain why many Christian theologians are much more cautious or restrictive about human cloning than leading Jewish rabbis, even though both traditions rely on the same general creation narrative.

In a public policy hearing, it is very difficult to explain these nuances and the assumptions behind interpretative selections and emphases. This is why religious discourse in a public context can sound dogmatic without intending to be such. However, certainly bioethicists who appeal to religious warrants must be prepared to address questions about both the internal coherence and the external relevance of the positions they advance.

In these respects, religious scholars and theologians are answerable to and accountable not only before their scholarly peers and their respective religious communities, but also before an audience of fellow citizens. In liberal political theory, it is these citizens who are the normative authorities. It is not the task of the theological ethicist to seek to win the assent of these public authorities to the moral authority of a sacred text. The tasks of answering and explicating are neither dogmatic nor evangelistic, but an appropriate form of public reasoning. This public reasoning involves the presentation of ideas that may (or may not) have influence without commanding authority.

It is also important to recognize that philosophical and secular ethics can be no less culpable of a form of authoritarianism. While it is commonplace to dismiss the normative weight religious communities may attribute to an account like Genesis on the grounds that it is antiquated and mythic, the philosophical foundations of ethics are no less rooted in mythic narratives. How is it, after all, that citizens come to be the moral authorities of the state? The response of liberal political theory is to construct a fictional state of nature or a veil of ignorance, out of which certain agreements are said to be arrived at mutually and by which the polity subsequently will be governed. In assessing diverse claims to moral authority, religious and secular narratives should be held to the same standard of historical reliability and credibility.

Fatalism

Perhaps the most constant objection in public discourse to biotechnology has been voiced through the metaphor of "playing God." The metaphor has a public resonance that is not limited to members of religious traditions; it is cited by nonreligious commentators to voice reservations about patenting and cloning.[24] The metaphor is a prime example of a religious concept that has influence but not political authority.

This kind of argumentation on biotechnology has been characterized as "fatalist," insofar as warnings about "playing God" or "manipulating nature" seem to imply that human beings are restricted from intervening in natural processes. The critique interprets fatalism to affirm that the task of human beings is submission to an order of nature that is divinely designed and therefore should be off-limits to human intervention and innovation. This entails acceptance that human life, destiny, and death are outside human control. Thus, human beings are rendered passive before powers that are arbitrary, capricious, and at times, abusive.

A striking literary portrait of the fatalist worldview is rendered in Albert Camus' *The Plague* through the character Paneloux. A priest and spiritual leader, Paneloux initially interprets the outbreak of plague within the city as a sign of divine judgment and punishment for sin, and calls upon his parishioners to do penance. Following the death of the child of the town magistrate, made horrific by an experimental medical remedy that embodies hope for a cure, but instead induces unrelieved convulsions, Paneloux comes to the conclusion that the deaths of the townspeople, and even of the child, are willed by God and that attempts to resist God's will are futile. The priest is eventually so paralyzed by this theology that he is unable to take any action at all, lest in doing so, God's will is violated.[25]

Paneloux embodies the logical extension of religious fatalism. A person must accept everything, good or ill, that comes his or her way as divinely ordained. The religious fatalist has no room for human choice or autonomy either to improve the human condition, or to prevent the situation from deteriorating into chaos. Alternately, if, as in the realm of medicine, procedures are used to intervene in natural processes for the purposes of control or mastery of disease and illness, the critique of religious fatalism maintains that it is then arbitrary to impose any restrictions on *any* subsequent interventions, such as human cloning, that are grounded solely in the will of God or the integrity of nature. Thus, ultimately, religious fatalism is deemed hostile to science, technology, and medicine, and philosophically opposed to choice and autonomy.[26] Having made a commitment to follow the will of God, the fatalist's only viable choice is passive submission.

When invoked uncritically in public discourse on biotechnology, the appeal to "playing God" risks these fatalist caricatures. However, the logic of fatalism is not recognizable in any tradition of religious thought. The language of "playing God" as Allen Verhey suggests, is not simply a warning, but also invokes a perspective."[27] The passion, imagination, and creativity presupposed in "play" elicits precisely those affective aspects of human nature that are critical to innovative scientific research and biotechnological breakthroughs. This affective character is simply neglected in the critique of fatalism and its relentless, rationalistic logic.

Paul Ramsey's summons that human beings should forgo playing God and instead learn what it means to be human,[28] while often interpreted as a warning and restrictive limit, can also be understood as a demand for recognition of a full embodied experience and meaning to the human person.[29] The human self is a complex interaction of body, spirit, and will; reason, consciousness, and emotion; nature, nurture, and supernature. By contrast, the critique of fatalism denies the complexity and opts instead for a misguided form of divine determinism. The crucial feature of religious thought is held to be the will, especially divine will, and thereby the core of the self is reduced to the possession or absence of capacities for making choices. However, this simply replicates religion in the image of the philosophical preoccupation with autonomy.

This fuller, embodied self of the religious traditions, in contrast to the disembodied mind of the philosophical traditions, views human beings as partners and participants with the divine in ordering human destiny. "Ordering," in contrast to "order," suggests a process that is dynamic and malleable, rather than rigid stasis, and one that is not at all compatible with passivity and submissiveness on the part of human beings.

Moreover, a fundamental dimension of the human experience of the divine is that of creator. Not only does this dimension elicit sentiments of gratitude and humility, but it also evokes an invitation for human beings to image the divine through imaginative and emotive creativity. Creativity is a "talent" (Matthew 25) that some human beings are gifted with and responsible for using to benefit themselves and their fellow humans. The expression of the talent or gift of creativity may be manifested in many different walks of life, including a propensity for scientific investigation and subsequent application in biotechnology. Thus, it is not only the worldview that is mistaken in the critique of religious fatalism, but also the portrait of the human self. The consequence is a critique with minimal credibility.

Divisiveness

Critics of religious discourse in public bioethics also cite fears of inflaming cultural division and polarization as grounds for an exclusionary discourse, an appeal validated by both historical and contemporary illustrations. Jeffrey Stout, for example, argues against a theological vindication for social morality on the following grounds: "The risks of reviving religious conflict like that of early modern Europe are too great."[30] As evidence for the probability of the risks of religious warfare in contemporary society, Stout points to examples "from Belfast to Beirut, from Teheran to Lynchburg, Virginia," as ample reason for concern.[31]

Thus, this argument runs, we should not think that the hateful emotions and violent actions unleashed by religious differences are remote from us in either time or space. According to some commentators, the age of religious wars of early modernity is different only in degree, not kind, from the "culture wars" of the late twentieth century. These contemporary wars are marked by the violence of language, intolerance toward difference, and an increasing social climate of incivility. Religious discourse, on this interpretation, is an agent of moral regress and social chaos, not the progress exemplified in modern science and biotechnology.[32]

This kind of perspective permeates bioethics pedagogy. A valuable teaching text begins its defense of a philosophical (i.e., rationalist) approach to bioethics by admonishing its readers that such an approach will enable them to "avoid violence" and "sidestep religion." This philosophic maneuvering is critical because conflict and religion are historically and *necessarily* connected: "[H]uman history illustrates all too well the futilities and dangers of relying solely upon religious principle to settle disputes between peoples of differing religious persuasions. A powerful motivation for engaging in philosophical argument about ethical matters . . . is the desire to avoid the deadlock and futility characteristic of religious disagreement."[33]

There are several points that may be offered in response to this challenge, but perhaps the place to begin is to acknowledge that the argument has some validity. It is not simply the blood shed for the cause of religion over the past half millennium in the West that bears out the point. Unlike the democratic liberal state, which affirms agnosticism toward the ultimate questions of life, religious traditions and communities embody perspectives on the good life for human beings and their communities. These cannot all be complementary, but instead must at times conflict. A vital question is whether there are resources within the religious traditions that can accommodate moral diversity and what Carter calls the autonomy of religions, or whether metaphysical differences must be enacted and resolved by coercion and even violence in the physical world.

Nevertheless, the risks to which Stout and others allude seem exaggerated and somewhat one-sided. If one part of the historical record must inevitably portray religion as a source of social oppression, in fairness that same record must also recognize religion as a source of liberation of the oppressed, whether from religious tyranny, economic slavery, or policies of segregation and discrimination. In this respect, Carter's observations of religious communities as "independent" voices of resistance are especially pertinent. If the fear of critics of religious discourse is regression to the anarchic Hobbesian state of nature, the remedy should not lie in the establishment of a secular leviathan of rationality, but rather in the granting of legitimized social space to religious communities to prevent tyranny without remedy.

These kinds of general considerations continue to surface in disputes over the ethics of biotechnology and the relevance of religious claims. There are historical and theoretical reasons that can be offered in support. But, in the context of the ethics of biotechnology, they fail to be convincing because they prefer simplification and sophistry to subtlety and sophistication. It needs to be shown, not simply asserted, that disagreement attributable to competing religious claims over the patenting of human genes or over cloning persons will necessarily issue in incivility and violence. Moreover, there seems to be a mistaken confidence in the leviathan of rationality that (1) it can be isolated in purest form from intuition, revelation, emotion, and other obstacles to clear-headed thinking, and (2) reliance on reason as the sole source of moral guidance provides a guarantee of agreement. Yet, the short history of biomedical ethics in the United States has illustrated that consensus is possible on concrete judgments even if there is disagreement on basic principles, and that fundamental theories of ethics that are often juxtaposed in opposition may nonetheless generate fairly similar intermediate principles and action guides.

I have examined four principal arguments against religious discourse that have emerged in ethical disputes about biotechnology, and most recently, about gene patenting and cloning. They are not without some basis. But, ultimately each argument tends to mistake what de Tocqueville referred to as religious influence as a grab for political authority by religious institutions. They fail to recognize that religious communities provide a valuable buffer zone in a secular state, as a source of resistance, and as a source of meaning in a society that is agnostic toward the questions of the good life and the good society. In the concluding section, I wish to turn to some of these themes of meaning embedded in patterns of religious discourse regarding biotechnology.

Biotechnology and Religious Meaning

It is part of both the appeal and temptation of biotechnology that we can find its accomplishments or prospects so astounding that we neglect to give attention to the social context within which the technology flourishes, and the human values it promotes or contradicts. Biotechnology may assume such a determining force in human culture that it becomes self-justifying and constitutes its own ends. Such a vision posed itself for Max Weber when, in the wake of the convergence of modern science, the industrial revolution, and economic capital at the beginning of the twentieth century, he warned that the questions of genuine human significance could get lost: "Natural science gives us an answer to the question of what we must do if we wish to master life technically. It leaves quite aside, or assumes for its purposes, whether we should and do wish to master life technically, and whether it ultimately makes sense to do so. . . . Science is meaningless because it gives no answer to our question, the only important question for us: What shall we do and how shall we live?"[34] Not only would we fail to answer such questions, but our capacity to even *raise* the questions would be dramatically inhibited by our quest for technological mastery and the consequent narrowing of moral vision. Thus, in the long run, Weber believed, we would find ourselves devolving into "specialists without spirit, sensualists without heart," trapped in a cage of our own technological making.[35]

One important role of autonomous religious communities is to retain their moral independence from technological specialization and mastery and infuse the debate over the ethics of biotechnology with a sense of spirit, heart, and meaning. That is, religious communities are positioned, and perhaps uniquely positioned in a liberal society, to attest that there is more at stake in the biotechnological revolution than creating a better crop through transgenic research or using animals as biofactories to express efficiently needed human proteins. These technological developments can profoundly shape our sense of who we are, and our relations with each other and the natural world. Religious communities cannot automatically accede to the authority of a technological worldview any more than they can affirm unswerving allegiance to the state; awareness of the biotechnological revolution must engage us in a process of exploring the boundaries and depths of human identity and destiny. In short, the technological quest opens up to the religious quest for meaning, purpose, and significance. By "meaning," I have reference to the ultimate questions of human experience, including our origins, nature, and destiny; our response to powers beyond our control, such as the genetic lottery of life; our finitude and fallibility; and our mortality. These questions are unavoidable if we are to approach the prospects of human-gene patenting or human cloning with scholarly seriousness and rigor. I want to present three claims about ultimacy and meaning that become particularly salient in the discussions about the theology and ethics of biotechnology: (1) the understanding of a child; (2) a narrative understanding of human life; and (3) human nature as creative.

Children: Choice or Gift?

Although de Tocqueville (and Carter) do not use the specific language, their discussion of the roles of religion in American civic life is compatible with recent discussion of the moral importance of intermediate communities. While much of the policy and philosophic ethical discussion on biotechnology has proceeded on an assumption that the primary stakeholders are individuals or couples (or an individual company) and the regulatory state, intermediate communities are, after all, the context for most of our meaningful life experiences. It is through participation in such communities, such as family, friendships, religious communities, and professional associations, that the relationship between the autonomous citizen and the authoritarian state is socially enacted and that values are transmitted and mediated. Moreover, such communities provide the most genuine, and most difficult, test of the integrity of our moral character, because our ethical convictions are always on display in these intimate and proximate relationships. Such communities thus have their own identity and integrity that influence how a question of social ethics and policy is framed and resolved; a moral vision that does not encompass the moral influence of these communities will be left with the minimalist resources of autonomy and utility, and examine the issues of biotechnology only from the standpoint of the impact of social (utility) restrictions or permissions on individual (scientific, reproductive, entrepreneurial) freedom or autonomy.

The moral influence of community, while certainly germane to discussions of gene patenting, is more prominent in the debate over human cloning, as religious voices have devoted sustained attention to the value of a child and the primacy of familial relationships. The current availability of reproductive technologies of various kinds, and the prospects of human clones in the near future, tends to make the child a human project, or as expressed by legal scholar John Robertson, a matter of "choice."[36] This position pointedly situates the child within the libertarian tradition of freedom, wherein decisions about whether the child will exist or not, and what characteristics, including gender, the child will have, are reflections of autonomous choice by the parents.

Of course, in reality, children are never completely products of deliberate and designed autonomous decisions. The child may instead be "a surprise," whose conception, gestational development, and birth evoke in parents basic sentiments of awe and wonder.[37] Religious discourse seeks to avoid reducing a child to an artifact of human choice and design through the language of "gift" and "mystery." Such language situates the child, not within traditions of personal autonomy, but rather within communal conventions and discourse about "gifts," that is, as entities that convey and embody personalization, foster mutuality and community, and encourage reciprocity.[38] Gifts represent a form of human exchange that cannot be reduced merely to market forces.

An understanding of the child as "gift" rather than "chosen project" makes intelligible the web of involuntary, unchosen responsibilities we experience that make up the moral infrastructure of an intermediate community. The principles of utility and autonomy can only offer an impoverished world of contractual commitments in which the child is an object through which we fulfill our own aims. Moreover, in the cloning process, the entity of *scientific* interest is the (somatic) cell, and the processes of cellular division; the child-to-be that is the outcome of the process is of secondary interest. Scientific and philosophical arguments in support of cloning have tended to emphasize the benefits of basic knowledge to researchers, or to potential treatments for human diseases, or to parents. Yet, as Daniel Callahan pointedly observes, "children in our world do not suffer from an absence of cloning."[39]

Moreover, the child continually reveals herself as resistant to our designs. Parents marvel at the child's physiological development, take joy in her projects, and become exasperated when their own moral authority is challenged or rejected. In all of this, the child is unfolded as mystery, beyond our ultimate control and understanding. Parents thereby learn of their limitations, and are reminded (certainly, by their children) of their fallibility.

Parenting involves profound moral commitments to preserving, nurturing, receptivity, and mutuality that are not adequately accommodated by moral frameworks of utility or autonomy. Such commitments are best sustained through the moral nexus of gifts rather than choice. Moreover, some religious traditions, particularly Judaism and Islam, give prominence to the importance of generational integrity and moral responsibilities that are rooted in genealogical lineage. This suggests a deep commitment to the kinds of ties that bind families together, as spouses, as parents, and as generations, and in turn why some theologians ultimately reject the prospects of human cloning on the grounds of "a good life in a family."[40] It is not a compelling counterargument to contend that current realities of familial life and relationships do not match theological idealism about the "good life in a family," because the political and philosophical framework of citizen and state as the primary moral relationship is itself a distortion of ordinary moral experience.

The Narrative Context

Religious arguments infuse spirit, heart, and meaning into debates on the ethics of biotechnology by situating methods such as gene patenting and cloning within their formative narratives. Religious narratives embody and express "mythic" dimensions of religious experience. I am here using "myth" not in the sense of a fabrication, but rather in a more academic sense of a story that (1) communicates a worldview or vision, (2) is revelatory for self-understanding, (3) sanctions models of behavior and moral norms, and (4) offers explanations for the eruption of evil or harm and the need for liberation.[41]

In this respect, it is perhaps no surprise that much of the discussion of religious communities about moral issues in general is given a narrative context. Moral norms are embedded in narratives, such as the norm of neighbor love in the Christian parable of the Good Samaritan and the norm of nonattachment in the Buddhist parable of the mustard seed. In the context of research on genetically engineered life forms, in which scientists, policymakers, bioentrepreneurs, and parents contemplate the creation of new life, religious traditions, whether Western, non-Western, or indigenous, are quite likely to draw analogues between biotechnology and their formative narratives of creation.[42]

As noted above, in Jewish and Christian traditions, religious arguments about cloning rely heavily on the creation stories related in Genesis. The narrative background establishes a particular view of self-understanding that is crucial to Jewish and Christian ethics on cloning, namely, that human beings are created in the "image of God" (*imago Dei*) and receive a mandate of dominion or stewardship. Religious traditions do differ over the meaning of the *imago Dei*, or in its application to the context of cloning human beings, but this claim about self-identity and understanding is a fundamental conviction of theological anthropology that addresses questions of ultimacy and meaning. And these convictions presuppose a background narrative and vision of the world.

Moreover, the narrative sanctions certain forms of behavior as acceptable based on moral norms. An account from the context of genetic analysis and Native American creation narratives is illustrative. For the past several years, a controversy with scientific, ethical, legal, and religious dimensions has developed over proposed DNA analysis of a hair sample retrieved in 1995 from "Kennewick Man," human remains believed to be some 9,500 years old that were uncovered in Washington State. The dispute is rooted in profoundly different views taken toward the human body and its parts, views that ultimately bear on the adequacy of genetic science within a culturally diverse society.

For the molecular scientist, the hair is a "sample," "evidence," a "key" to advancing scientific knowledge of cultural anthropology. The hair is easily separable from the person whose hair it once was. For the native communities, however, hair is composed of the fundamental elements of the world—male rain, female rain, and the moisture of clouds—as delineated in the cultural myths of creation. Hair represents mind and thought, and is the embodiment of lifelong knowledge. This narrative generates a communal norm that hair is not to be cut, except under certain well-defined ritual circumstances, or unless the hair is bound up in a symbolic pattern. Hair thus cannot be severed from the person, and the narrative ways of life of a culture and people. To subject the hair to DNA testing is an act with cosmic consequences; a patent is sacrilege.

My point is that hair is not always or only "hair." Even a single strand that may invite scientific analysis at a molecular level is, within a different cultural context, a richly layered expression of self, history, and meaning. This phenomenon is a variation of what Nelkin and Lindee refer to as the "DNA mystique": A gene is not only a gene in the context of scientific and public narratives, but has also become the new marker for the "soul," or the human essence.[43]

An important question in this context concerns self-location within the body: "*Where* am I in my body?" Some possible responses, reflecting different cultural traditions, might be, "behind the eyes," or "within the chest," or even "in the womb." Yet, the question of self-location may not even be intelligible within certain native cultures, such as the traditional Navajo, whose understanding of self precludes the reductionism pervasive in contemporary biomedical science. The Navajo have an extended sense of personhood: Personality is indivisible, residing as a whole in each of the parts.[44] Thus, traditional Navajos might respond to the question, "I am *throughout* the body."

The formative narratives of this traditional culture invest body parts with enormous mythological significance; particular parts of the body, such as the afterbirth or the umbilical cord, are held to possess the ability to produce consequences in the world and for others. The umbilical cord, for example, can influence a child's inclinations, occupation, and relationships. The tissues of pre-birth life sustenance are not post-birth organic refuse, or a rich source of stem cells for clinical research, or a potential "gold mine" for commercial development. In short, they are not *re-sources* for use by others, but *sources* of life and knowledge. Among health care facilities that provide services to the Navajo, it is customary as a sign of respect for these beliefs that, subsequent to birth, the placenta and umbilical cord are returned to the family for disposal (usually by burial) rather than requesting consent for the use of the tissue in medical research or educational projects.[45]

This sense of integration of self throughout the entire body implicitly extends to genes, and the language of "gene" is used among acculturated Navajo. Amongst traditional Navajo, genetic relationships are embedded in "blood" lines. The Navajo understand personal identity to be constituted by four types of blood, derived from four clans: maternal, paternal, maternal grandfather, and paternal grandfather. These different forms of blood, or clans, influence the development and functioning of the basic bodily systems.[46] Within this worldview, then, something that seems as innocuous as a request for a blood draw has enormous symbolic repercussions. It is to initiate an inquiry not into a biological entity, but rather to probe a person's culture and history, and therefore the personal identity of a Navajo.

In Navajo narratives (and those of many religious traditions), wind or breath is the animating life force. The prints of the fingers and toes bear the marks of this animating force. The whorls on the tips of fingers and toes (and on the back of the head) that distinguish us from each other are, for the traditional Navajo, a sign of our commonality. The whorls are the marks on the body surface that locate the entrance and departure of the animating winds of life. Those on our toes serve to anchor us firmly in the ground, the body of Mother Earth. Those on our fingers tie us to Father Sky. In this way, we are able to walk upright through the power of the winds without falling down.

My principal claim from these illustrations is that the formative narratives of religious communities are an important source for insight into the moral meaning of biotechnology. They disclose worldviews and patterns of life, present modes of self-understanding, and reveal moral norms that are especially valuable in moral perception. When such narratives are invoked in public discourse, they stimulate public imagination by posing alternative understandings and meanings on genetic research or cloning. They can enhance moral deliberation by illuminating how a gene sample can raise profound questions of human origins and human identity.

It is of significance that for most religious communities, biotechnology is narratively contextualized through stories of creation or of human beginnings. Put another way, practices such as genetic analysis, patenting, or cloning seldom invoke narratives of redemption or liberation. This is to say that, while biotechnology may be viewed as providing alternative ways of enhancing the quality of human life, or of bringing life into the world, such practices are at best morally optional, rather than morally required. Nonetheless, as scientific techniques have become more efficient and effective, some religious thinkers have begun to understand biotechnology within narratives of eschatology or human destiny, as an expression of an evolving human nature.

Creating Human Destiny

Even for religious traditions that situate biotechnological developments within narratives of creation, there remains a question about whether creation is *normative*. Do human beings "look backward" for moral guidance and to culturally regain or approximate a paradise lost? This perspective, involving a "recovery" of human nature, is certainly important to arguments presented by many religious thinkers, and by and large, it leads to cautious theological assessments of the ethics of biotechnology. It no less opens up these traditions to the critique of fatalism delineated above.

However, another theological interpretation is possible, one that emphasizes a "discovery" of human nature and an openness about human destiny. This perspective begins from the insight that it is through imagination and creativity that we engage the authentically human and reflect the image of the divine in interactions with other persons and with nature. This warrants not only aesthetic expression but also a sanction for the research and use of various technologies to improve the human condition. The human gaze is thereby redirected from a backward look to a forward vision, in which creation is understood not as static and fixed at a particular time, but as a dynamic *process*, within which normative humanity and human destiny evolves over time and is continually re-created. Creation is an ongoing process, a continual creation (*continuo creatio*) to which human beings are called to active participation.

Such an account, which is most prominent in liberal Protestant thought, can accommodate, permit, or even encourage applications of biotechnology.[47] This includes support for genetic research and patenting, and perhaps cloning of human beings as an expression of human creativity to the extent that the particular technique promotes human welfare and dignity. While biotechnology is still not seen in the light of redemption or liberation, it is nonetheless not constrained so significantly by an interpretation of nature that is essentially "fixed" from creation. The moral meaning of biotechnology is therefore derived from an understanding of human possibilities (in partnership with the divine) and theologies of hope.

This paradigm shift is illustrated in some recent theological writing on human cloning. Lutheran theologian Ted Peters, for example, maintains that, "on distinctively theological grounds no good reason for proscribing human cloning can be mustered."[48] Peters does not argue that there are "no good reasons" at all that would limit cloning, but rather that these cannot be generated from within a theological position. However, even these reasons (which have to do with parental expectations and the dignity of children) provide only a basis for "caution" about cloning, not proscription. Ethically, it is important to recognize that reliance on a theological anthropology of evolving humanity and an open-ended human destiny, rather than on one of created human nature, dramatically shifts the moral burden of proof. That burden shifts from those who wish to proceed with cloning to those who seek its restraint and/or prohibition. In general, biotechnology is presumed innocent until the infliction of actual harm can be substantiated, rather than guilty until substantive benefit can be shown.

I want to claim, however, that Peters is mistaken in suggesting that concern for the dignity of children cannot rest on grounds that are distinctive to theological claims. Some recent work within philosophical bioethics has begun to give attention to an ethics of family life.[49] However, as valuable as these discussions are, they remain peripheral to the central concerns and presuppositions of philosophical bioethics, which as noted, give moral primacy to the relation between the citizen and the state, and to the principles of respect for autonomy and utility. The dignity of children is at best a derivative claim, in part because the family is a historical anachronism in the dominant tradition of liberal individualism. Indeed, the notion of intermediate communities is a philosophical anomaly for this tradition. Religious voices, by contrast, begin with relationships between selves, rather than the solitary self, and speak of the child as a "gift" rather than a "choice" or "product." There are, then, distinctive theological motivations and warrants for the concept of the dignity of children. The language of "gift" resonates within the broader culture and has influence while not claiming authority.[50]

While the theological endeavor to discover human nature is to be commended for emphasizing openness to creativity and technological innovation, a more general problem is that it does not seem to offer any grounds for limitations. After all, if normative humanity is undergoing continual re-creation and interpretation, then the concepts of "human welfare" or "human dignity" are themselves rendered conceptually fluid and thereby problematic. The theological emphasis on a creative human destiny, while avoiding a static standard of the normatively human, doesn't seem to be able to generate any viable standard in its place.

Projects of our creativity and imagination, including technological innovations, are subject to the constraints of finitude and fallibility. We have limited capacities to predict or control the outcomes of courses of action that we initiate, and it is difficult (and some would argue, impossible) for us to be morally disinterested in these actions to the point of being able to offer valid ethical assessments. Secular, theological, and popular literature are replete with examples of where creativity was not balanced with or checked by awareness of finitude and the possibilities of fallibility: Almost every cultural tradition, including modern science, has its version of the Promethean myth. If our human propensities for aspiration and pretension are theologically downplayed, then narratives from Genesis, or popular literature such as *Frankenstein*, *Brave New World*, or *Jurassic Park*, remind us that what is created can ultimately rebel and consume the creator with catastrophic consequences. In this respect, it is difficult to avoid the questions posed about human identity in the context of considering technology that inevitably redefines what it means to be who we are.

Conclusion

This essay has sought to display points of both contact and conflict between traditions of religious ethics and public policy in debates over biotechnology, including gene patenting and human cloning. I have argued for a model of religious community and discourse that is centered on the concept of "meaningful resistance." In this model, it is possible to discern a unity amongst religious pluralism with respect to the kinds of questions asked of biotechnology. These questions can and do have influence in public moral discourse, but they do not and should not command political authority. It is through raising questions and critiques of biotechnology that religious traditions express resistance to dominant institutions in social life, including science, industry, and the state. The autonomy or independence of religions from these institutions enables such questions to be asked with integrity to the core values of the tradition.

Moreover, these issues of resistance express deep themes of meaning for religious communities. At stake in the context of genetic analysis and patenting, and in the cloning of human beings, are matters of how we ought to live our lives, and about human nature, identity, and destiny. Biotechnology brings to the forefront important assumptions about understandings of children and parenting, and about our nature as persons in communities constituted by formative narratives. As the liberal state has adopted an attitude of agnosticism about the good life for persons in their communities, religious traditions make a distinctive contribution to the policy process over the ethics of biotechnology by posing as central these themes of meaning. In this context, inevitably, religious discourse will have influence beyond the boundaries of a particular religious community.

NOTES

1. President's Commission for the Study of Ethical Problems in Medicine and Biomedical and Behavioral Research, *Splicing Life: A Report on the Social and Ethical Issues of Genetic Engineering with Human Beings* (Washington, D.C.: U.S. Government Printing Office, 1982).

2. R. C. Lewontin, "The Confusion over Cloning," *The New York Review of Books* (October 23, 1997): 18–23, at 22; G. E. Pence, *Who's Afraid of Human Cloning?* (New York: Rowman and Littlefield Publishers, Inc., 1998), pp. 34–35.

3. Leroy Walters, "Religion and the Renaissance of Medical Ethics in the United States: 1965–1975," in *Theology and Bioethics: Exploring the Foundations and Frontiers*, ed. Earl E. Shelp (Boston: D. Reidel Publishing Company, 1985), pp. 3–16.

4. James F. Childress, "The Challenges of Public Ethics: Reflections on NBAC's Report," *Hastings Center Report* 27, no. 5 (1997): 9–11.

5. L. Shiner, "The Meanings of Secularization," in *Secularization and the Protestant Prospect*, ed. James F. Childress and D. B. Harned (Philadelphia: Westminster Press, 1970), pp. 30–42.

6. Kent Greenawalt, *Religious Convictions and Political Choice* (New York: Oxford University Press, 1988), pp. 14–48.

7. Pence, *Who's Afraid*, p. 35.

8. Stephen L. Carter, *The Culture of Disbelief: How American Law and Politics Trivialize Religious Devotion* (New York: Basic Books, 1993), pp. 23–43.

9. Alexis de Tocqueville, *Democracy in America*, ed. J. P. Mayer (Garden City, N.Y.: Anchor Books, 1969), pp. 298–99.

10. de Tocqueville, *Democracy in America*, p. 298.

11. de Tocqueville, *Democracy in America*, p. 292.

12. Carter, *The Culture of Disbelief*, pp. 36–37.

13. Carter, *The Culture of Disbelief*, pp. 37–41.

14. Carter, *The Culture of Disbelief*, p. 40.

15. H. Tristram Engelhardt, Jr., "Looking for God and Finding the Abyss: Bioethics and Natural Theology," in *Theology and Bioethics: Exploring the Foundations and Frontiers*, ed. Earl E. Shelp (Boston: D. Reidel Publishing Company, 1985), pp. 79–91.

16. James F. Childress, remarks at Project Meeting on Religion and Biotechnology, The Hastings Center, November 1997.

17. Jonathan D. Moreno, *Deciding Together: Bioethics and Moral Consensus* (New York: Oxford University Press, 1995).

18. Martin Benjamin, *Splitting the Difference: Compromise and Integrity in Ethics and Politics* (Lawrence: University of Kansas Press, 1990); Max Weber, "Politics as a Vocation; Science as a Vocation," in Weber, *From Max Weber: Essays*

in Sociology, ed. H. H. Gerth and C. W. Mills (New York: Oxford University Press, 1958), pp. 77–156.

19. Joseph Fletcher, *Morals and Medicine* (Boston: Beacon Press, 1954).

20. Lewontin, "The Confusion over Cloning," p. 23.

21. Pence, *Who's Afraid*, pp. 63, 142.

22. Courtney S. Campbell and J. Woolfrey, "Norms and Narratives: Religious Reflections on the Human Cloning Controversy," *Journal of Biolaw and Business* 1, no. 3 (1998): 8–20.

23. Allen Verhey, *The Great Reversal: Ethics and the New Testament* (Grand Rapids, Mich.: Eerdmans Pub. Co., 1984).

24. E. R. Gold, *Body Parts: Property Rights and the Ownership of Human Biological Materials* (Washington, D.C.: Georgetown University Press, 1996); A. Kimbrell, *The Human Body Shop: The Engineering and Marketing of Life* (San Francisco: Harper Collins Publishers, 1993).

25. Albert Camus, *The Plague* (New York: Vintage Books, 1972).

26. Pence, *Who's Afraid*, pp. 122–29.

27. Allen Verhey, "Playing God and Invoking a Perspective," *Journal of Medicine and Philosophy* 20 (1995): 347–64.

28. Paul Ramsey, *Fabricated Man: The Ethics of Genetic Control* (New Haven, Conn.: Yale University Press, 1970), p. 138.

29. Ramsey, *Fabricated Man*.

30. Jeffrey Stout, *Ethics After Babel: The Languages of Morals and Their Discontents* (Boston: Beacon Press, 1988), p. 223.

31. Stout, *Ethics after Babel*, p. 223.

32. Childress, remarks at Project Meeting on Religion and Biotechnology, The Hastings Center, Garrison, N.Y., November 1997.

33. A. Ridley, *Beginning Bioethics: A Text with Integrated Readings* (New York: St. Martin's Press, 1998), p. 6.

34. Weber, "Politics as a Vocation," p. 144.

35. Max Weber, *The Protestant Ethic and the Spirit of Capitalism* (New York: Scribner, 1958).

36. John A. Robertson, *Children of Choice: Freedom and the New Reproductive Technologies* (Princeton, N.J.: Princeton University Press, 1994).

37. Paul Ramsey, "On In Vitro Fertilization," in *On Moral Medicine: Theological Perspectives in Medical Ethics*, ed. Stephen E. Lammers and Allen Verhey (Grand Rapids, Mich.: Eerdmann's Publishing Co., 1987), pp. 339–44, at 344.

38. Paul Camenisch, "Gift and Gratitude in Ethics," *Journal of Religious Ethics* 9 (1981): 1–34; Thomas H. Murray, *The Worth of a Child* (Berkeley: University of California Press, 1996).

39. Daniel Callahan, "Cloning: The Work Not Done," *Hastings Center Report* 27, no. 5 (1997): 18–20, at 19.

40. Allen Verhey, "Theology After Dolly," *Christian Century* (19–26 March 1997): 285–86.

41. J. C. Livingston, *Anatomy of the Sacred* (New York: Macmillan Publishing Company, 1989).

42. Campbell and Woolfrey, "Norms and Narratives."

43. Dorothy Nelkin and M. Susan Lindee, *The DNA Mystique: The Gene as a Cultural Icon* (New York: Freeman, 1995).

44. M. T. Schwarz, *Molded in the Image of Changing Woman: Navajo Views on the Human Body and Personhood* (Tucson: University of Arizona Press, 1997).

45. W. L. Freeman, "The Role of Community in Research with Stored Tissue Samples," unpublished manuscript, p. 16.

46. Schwarz, *Molded in the Image.*

47. Ted Peters, *Playing God? Genetic Determinism and Human Freedom* (New York, Routledge, 1997); Ronald Cole-Turner, *The New Genesis: Theology and the Genetic Revolution* (Louisville, Ky.: Westminster/John Knox Press, 1993).

48. Ted Peters, "Cloning Shock: A Theological Reaction," in *Human Cloning: Religious Responses*, ed. Ronald Cole-Turner (Louisville, Ky.: Westminster/John Knox Press, 1997), pp. 12–24.

49. Thomas H. Murray, "Gifts of the Body and the Needs of Strangers," *Hastings Center Report* 17, no. 2 (1987): 30–38; Hilde Lindemann Nelson and James Lindemann Nelson, *The Patient in the Family: An Ethics of Medicine and Families* (New York: Routledge, 1995).

50. Childress, remarks at Project Meeting on Religion and Biotechnology, The Hastings Center, November 1997.

B. Andrew Lustig

Human Cloning and Liberal Neutrality: Why We Need to Broaden the Public Dialogue

One often hears that the claims of religious communities are epistemologically privileged, and therefore inaccessible to others who do not share the faith that undergirds such tenets. That notion of epistemological inaccessibility is nowhere more in evidence than in the contentious debates of bioethics, where religious worldviews are often viewed as parochial, necessarily divisive, and therefore incapable of contributing to the shared warrants for public policy.[1]

Such theoretical dismissal of religious arguments from the public square, however, is belied by the function of religious voices in many policy debates. There are two obvious rejoinders to such a caricature of religion in the policy process—one, an appeal to the moral logic at work in religious arguments, and the second, an appeal to the actual history of policy formation on disputed issues in bioethics. First, to disqualify expressly religious voices from the public square, one must assume that religious arguments, because they are framed in particular ways, lack affinities with arguments not so grounded. This assumption, however, overlooks the significant place, in many religious traditions, for the accessibility of religiously based arguments to others who are not persuaded by underlying faith claims. Consider, for example, appeals in Roman Catholic teaching to natural law as a shared basis for moral reflections, on matters of both personal and social morality. Consider the distinction in Judaism between the commandments binding on Jewish believers and the broader "Noahide" commandments meant to govern the behavior of both Jews and Gentiles. Consider, in Islam, appeals made to the shared moral code among Muslims, Jews, and Christians, all deemed to be "people of the Book." Thus, even a cursory acquaintance with religious worldviews indicates that the parochialism and divisiveness imputed to such perspectives are not necessary features. Second, in the context of policy debates in the United States, the nature and scope of First Amendment protections are often interpreted in ways that would disqualify religious voices from the public square. Again, that interpretation is demonstrably false. Instead, what amounts to an overlapping consensus—despite differing theological, philosophical, and political values held by those who reach agreement—serves to ground significant policy choices, in bioethics and elsewhere. The often polemical effort to exclude religious voices from policy debates confuses the *process* of public discussion—where the views of particular communities, including religious ones, may exert legitimate influence—with the *justification* of policy choices, where parochial appeals may indeed be inappropriate.

Recent debates regarding the possibility of human cloning exemplify the above set of concerns. In this chapter, I will not develop in detail the expressly religious arguments offered against cloning on their own terms. Rather, after briefly reviewing recent religious discussion, I will consider the possibilities of drawing *parallels* between religious and nonreligious arguments against human cloning. I do so for two reasons, one theoretical, the other practical. As a matter of theory, while religious arguments are indeed distinctive in their fundamental warrants, I will suggest that their character as arguments is not unique, but often functionally equivalent to many nonreligious perspectives. Thus, if the latter are not deemed illegitimate in political debate—and usually, if cast in secular language, they are not—neither should religious appeals.

As a practical matter, in the context of the discussion about human cloning, I believe that certain nonreligious appeals function *analogously* to expressly religious appeals. Hence, the insistence by many commentators (including members of the National Bioethics Advisory Commission [hereinafter NBAC])[2] that religious insights be "translated" into a language accessible to secular hearers seems equally well directed at arguments that, while not expressly religious, involve appeals to moral or aesthetic values that are framed in particularistic fashion. For example, in relation to new developments in reproductive technologies, secular appeals to the "wonder" of procreation, secular fears raised about "illicit tampering" with human nature, or secular concerns about broader social attitudes concerning family life may share the problem of "translatability" with expressly religious appeals. In both instances, those who raise broad concerns about values or interests that cannot be immediately and unambiguously specified as obvious harms to particular individuals are left at a clear disadvantage. Indeed, their concerns are often dismissed as merely "symbolic" or "speculative," as if, apparently, by such descriptions, forms of reasoning other than economic calculations of cost and benefit cannot play a role in the crafting of public policy.

What is less often noted, in this insistence that particularistic arguments must be translated into a moral Esperanto accessible to all hearers, is that the burden of proof for such translation has been assigned, without argument, to those who *speak* in the public square, rather than those who *listen*. It is not obvious, in any version of democratic theory with which I am familiar, why this should be so. Indeed, this burden of translation incumbent on speakers, rather than listeners, of the political word, far from being a requirement of public discourse, instead reflects the impoverished view of policy formation reflected in much bioethics discussion. In moving toward that conclusion, through the prism of the debate on human cloning, I will suggest that certain themes in recent communitarian thought, if taken seriously, can offer useful correctives to the narrow methodological and theoretical commitments of much recent political theory. I will then conclude with a few remarks about a wider understanding of public reasoning which, by not assuming the priority of unfettered individual autonomy, can more readily consider and incorporate appeals to broader aesthetic, moral, or religiously based concerns as important elements of public discourse and policy formation. That understanding entertains a more robust vision of both politics and policy formation, one that takes note of the various *levels* at which public discussion occurs, the various *forms* of discourse available at different levels and in different settings, and the various *publics* served by different sources of authority, only some of which will be reflected in policy and law.

The Liberal Neutrality Thesis Applied to the Prospect of Human Cloning

There are two core notions of what is called the "liberal neutrality thesis" (hereinafter LNT). Empirically, the LNT acknowledges the diverse values held by individuals in pluralistic democracies. From that empirical judgment, a political strategy of accommodation follows. According to the LNT, it is inappropriate to assume, much less to invoke, a "thick" or robust understanding of human good that can direct policy choices. That strategy of accommodation has led to an emphasis, especially in the Rawlsian literature, on the necessity of a "thin theory" of the good, one that is minimal but sufficient to form the basic institutions of society.[3]

In the wake of Dr. Ian Wilmut's announcement of apparently success-ful mammalian cloning—and the rush of subsequent developments—many concerns have been raised about human cloning that involve particularistic appeals, including the speculative but plausible future harms associated with cloning as but another step toward a "brave new world" that many find troubling. According to the LNT, a thick or substantive version of human good is difficult to specify in a way that can illuminate and direct pluralistic policy choice. *A fortiori*, harm—as the deprivation of a substantive good—will be equally if not more difficult to articulate with precision. For example, the NBAC, in its report *Cloning Human Beings*, achieved consensus for its current recom-mendations solely on the basis of a form of harm obvious to all current observers—given current safety risks, the potential for *physical* harm posed to an individual born as the result of somatic cell nuclear transfer.[4]

In light of the agnosticism of the LNT, the narrow basis of the NBAC consensus is unsurprising. For the range of harms that can be specified within some appeal to a substantive vision of the good will necessarily be limited, probably to such obvious instances of physical harm. Other concerns—especially imprecise appeals to such notions as "offensiveness" or "repugnance"[5]—or criticisms that invoke the lan-guage of "intuitions" or "anxieties"—will, given LNT premises, be of marginal relevance to policy discussion. And note again: The difficulties posed here by the LNT about the appropriate basis of pluralistic policy are not directed to religious versus secular reasons. Rather, the require-ments of the LNT neutrality thesis apply to all epistemologically privi-leged appeals, whatever their provenance.

Functional Parallels between Religious and Secular Arguments

Religious Arguments

Those who oppose the prospect of human cloning on expressly religious grounds do so by invoking a number of theological themes and values. As I said above, I will not explore those themes or their applications here in depth or detail. (Indeed, I would suggest that significant work remains to make many of these arguments theologically compelling on their own terms.) However, drawing from the NBAC report, I will provide a brief overview of key theological understandings as a prelude to comparing such arguments with those that oppose human cloning on nonreligious grounds.[6] I offer the comparison with a particular aim: to show that religiously informed objections may functionally parallel certain secular arguments in ways that call into question the adequacy of the LNT as a template for public policy discussion and formation.

The NBAC report, in its chapter on religious perspectives, discusses several major theological themes and concerns relevant to an assessment of human cloning. The following five are especially prominent. First, especially in Judaism and Christianity, the distinctiveness of humans is ascribed to their being created in the image of God. Second, as creatures made in God's image, humans are called to exercise responsible dominion over nature. Human dominion is variously described as stewardship, partnership, or "created co-creation." These themes, in turn, lead to various assessments of the legitimate nature and scope of human interventions into nature (including human nature) in pursuit of human benefit or betterment. Third, religious discussions appeal to the central value of human dignity, based again upon an understanding of human beings as imagers of God. Religious opposition to human cloning based on appeals to human dignity may involve different dimensions of that value: psychological threats to individuality, concerns about sanctity of life in relation to the status of cloned embryos and fetuses, and/or worries about objectification and commodification in relation to sources of genetic material and cloned "offspring." Fourth, broad concerns are voiced about the implications of cloning for the institution of parenting, attitudes toward children, and the possible impact of human cloning on our understanding of intergenerational relations. Fifth, some religious commentators, setting the prospect of human cloning within the larger context of allocation questions, have questioned the justice of pursuing human cloning research in light of other more pressing needs.[7] In light of such fundamental concerns, the NBAC report concluded that "most religious thinkers who recommend public policies on cloning humans propose either a ban or restrictive legislation."[8] As a summary observation, it seems fair to observe that the majority of religious commentators on human cloning have assessed it in either thoroughly negative, or cautiously circumscribed, terms.

Secular Concerns Raised about Human Cloning

In addition to religiously framed arguments, many thoughtful secular commentators have also expressed anxieties about the prospect of human cloning. A first impetus for such secular anxiety is identified by the NBAC as the basis of its current consensus recommendations: the serious risk of physical harm to individuals born as the result of somatic nuclear cell transfer experiments, given the state of current research knowledge. Granted, this basis for opposition is quite provisional. Much as with early debates regarding in-vitro fertilization, NBAC's assumption is that animal experimentation will be likely to resolve the issue of what constitutes an "acceptable" risk in pursuit of progeny.

A second set of concerns raised about human cloning implicates our fundamental perspectives on "human nature" itself as a category of both personal morality and public policy. While technological optimists might view us as infinitely malleable, a number of secular critics of cloning appeal to an intuitive sense of "natural" or "appropriate" limits to reproductive options and practices, or to a natural judgment of human cloning as "offensive" or "repugnant."[9]

A third concern appeals to the history of eugenics in cautioning us against the dangers of abuse if we continue, without limits, upon the road to genetic enhancement as a desirable goal for couples. While cloning is, properly speaking, not enhancement, but replication of an extant genome, it involves a "new way" of specifying reproduction according to human desire and design, and raises similar issues, by the spirit, if not the letter, of its technique.

A fourth set of concerns involves attitudes ranging from cautious skepticism to outright fear of new forms of technology. In this respect, cloning, and other forms of reproductive experimentation, evoke attitudes prompted by concerns about technology more generally. We are, especially at the turn of this new century, aware of the mixed blessings of technology, and have learned to be wary of excessive, even utopian, claims of progress from technological optimists. Hence, developments in reproductive technology evince our larger sense of "distrust" about the mixed results of technology. But genetic technologies also prompt reactions that are different in degree, if not in kind, from our more general distrust of technology, because of the sense that we are, with a directness and immediacy not heretofore imagined, choosing to manipulate ourselves in new ways, with results that cannot be clearly foreseen. Thus cloning, as the duplication of a genotype that has already occurred, while not "genetic engineering" in the strict sense, resonates emotionally with other more direct forms of manipulation of the genotype because of the purposiveness of such duplication. While some may note, correctly, that genetically identical twins "naturally" occur, that seems a curious argument to invoke in a vacuum. There is much in nature that occurs that we would not wish to mimic as an object of human choice and design. The concern here relates not to the "uniqueness" of the result, but the appropriateness of our choice toward that end.

Closely associated with some of the above concerns are what might be called the "Frankenstein factor," a sense that despite intentions we initially deem legitimate, things will go awry, that our genies (or monsters), once loosed, will run amuck. There is also what has been described as the "yuk factor," the sense that we are tinkering and tampering in ways that are "creepy," that make us feel "out of place."[10]

There are also secular concerns raised regarding issues of social justice and commodification, which are relevant not only to cloning but to other forms of new reproductive technologies and practices. Insofar as such technologies are made available only to those who can afford them, they are likely to increase disparities between "haves" and "have nots," not only within nations but between developed and developing countries. Moreover, the prospect of human cloning poses particular issues of objectification and commodification if, indeed, at some point, "desirable" genotypes are made available for subsequent cloning, in a manner that is different in degree, if not in kind, from the commodification of gametes.

There are doubtless other nonreligious concerns that might be invoked in arguing against the prospect of human cloning. But however much one expands the list, what such concerns reveal, perhaps less individually than taken together, is a sense of *collective unease* with the perils that the prospect of human cloning presents. A particular argument may appear inadequate to counter the putative force of the claim that, when "safety issues" are resolved, reproductive rights should be extended to cloning as yet another option. Yet, these many other concerns— both religious and secular—might, when *considered together*, counter simplistic assertions of reproductive rights. Indeed, I believe there exists a "common ground" that can be identified between religious and nonreligious objections, and that such religious and secular parallels reveal something akin to a notion of the "common good," which might serve to moderate the excessive individualism at work in much recent discussion of new reproductive technologies and practices.

The Possibilities of Convergence between Religious and Secular Arguments against Cloning

Of particular interest, from the perspective of what constitutes appropriate public policy, is the tendency by proponents of cloning to narrow their moral focus to calculations of cost and benefit, and to reject appeals to moral intuition, moral vision, and moral imagination as relevant features of our pluralistic discourse. Yet, the paucity of our common language here reflects, I think, an abandonment of the very vocabulary we need to make sense of the implications of human cloning as a serious possibility—its implications for practices of parenting, its implications for our understanding of the nature of human nature, and its underscoring of our need for a renewal of a collective moral language, a language of the common good that allows policy space for the voicing of broader, less easily specifiable concerns, whether these are framed in religious or secular terms. I submit that clear affinities can be found between a number of religious and secular arguments made against human cloning, and that such overlapping values can provide resources for richer and more substantive conversation in the crafting of appropriate public policy. I now consider two such correspondences—religious and secular arguments about psychological threats to the individuality of the human clone, and concerns expressed about the attitudes constitutive of parenting as a practice.

Implications of cloning for our understanding of embodied individuality. For many thinkers, cloning would, as a deliberate choice, pose unacceptable threats to the psychological well-being of the clone himself or herself. Although proponents of cloning dismiss these concerns as merely speculative or symbolic, the holistic perspective at work in both religious and secular understandings helps to clarify how cloning might well undermine the dignity of the person who is cloned.

Human beings, religionists say, are made in the image of God. This language means that, as creatures, we are unitary wholes, composed of body, soul, and spirit. We are not immortal souls in bodies, as if our bodies are incidental to our essential selves. Nor are our "spirits" (or, for secularists, our "psyches") reducible to our bodies. Any form of reductionism that would explain away our spiritual or psychic nature by reducing it to an epiphenomenon, reducible to the laws of physics and biology, is equally unacceptable. A holistic understanding of the human person—religious or secular—sees us as unitary wholes. On the one hand, holism would not fall prey to genetic reductionism; thus a human clone, though a younger genetic twin, would not be the same person. Nature *and* nurture, after all, are both at work in the formation of our personalities. Any crude notion that replicating a genotype would be replicating a person would be mistaken. On the other hand, holism would not trivialize the importance of our physical selves to our well-being as persons. Thus we cannot make light of how such planned replication would be likely to affect the person cloned. The notion that such harms are "merely speculative," as the supporters of cloning contend, does not diminish their force. While the clone would be a distinct individual, we know quite well that our genetic and phenotypic differences reinforce our sense of distinctive identity. It seems quite likely that human clones would face greater difficulties in establishing a unique sense of self. It seems equally likely that those who replicate human clones would burden them with prior expectations, thus infringing on their freedom to become unique individuals. Why, otherwise, would cloning seem so desirable for those who espouse it as a way to replicate gifted individuals?

Begetting or making? Implications of cloning for parenting.
Anglican theologian Oliver O'Donovan, in his 1984 book entitled *Begotten or Made?* viewed cloning as a perverse expression of the tendency to objectify children as products of our own will, different in degree, if not in kind, from other forms of assisted reproduction. With cloning, we specify in advance a full human genotype, we close ourselves to the usual novelty of sexual begetting, and we impose our intentions upon a child in a new and revolutionary way. "The development of cloning," O'Donovan said, "will be a demonstration, if it occurs, that mankind does have the awesome technical power to exchange the humanity which God has given him for something else, to treat natural humanity itself as a raw material for constructing a form of life that is not natural humanity but is an artificial development out of humanity."[11]

In O'Donovan's judgment, the process of cloning would fundamentally alter the relationship between parent and child. Unlike other forms of assisted reproduction, which simply facilitate the ordinary process of conception, with replication the perspective shifts. While in natural procreation, a child is begotten by virtue of what we *are*, cloning gives existence to a being not by what we are but by what we intend and design.

While O'Donovan frames this distinction in theological terms, it also resonates with commentators who speak in more broadly humanistic fashion. For example, Leon Kass, in a number of writings, develops the same distinction. Most recently, he has expressed his concern in these terms:

> Human cloning would . . . represent a giant step toward turning begetting into making, procreation into manufacture . . . a process already begun

with in vitro fertilization and genetic testing of embryos. With cloning, not only is the process in hand, but the total genetic blueprint of the cloned individual is selected and determined by human artisans. . . . [W]e here would be taking a major step into making man himself simply another of the man-made things . . . [t]o be homogenized by our rationalized technique according to the subjective prejudices of the day.[12]

"Getting the point" of the distinction between begetting and making—whether argued on religious or secular grounds—requires more than the calculus of reproductive autonomy and preference satisfaction. It requires habits of heart and imagination, and a reflective wisdom that moves beyond mere intellectual debate. It requires a willingness to discern the larger potential—for good and ill—of our own longings, only some of which redound to the benefit of our children and ourselves. Religious ethicist Allen Verhey captures the point quite well:

> If we see children as achievements, as products, then the "quality control" approach appropriate to technology will gradually limit our options to choosing either a perfect child or a dead child. Our capacity as parents to provide the sort of uncalculating care and nurture that evokes the trust of children will be diminished. If we would cherish children as begotten, not made, as gifts, not products, then we will not be hospitable to cloning.[13]

To appreciate the collective force of such concerns (however imprecise they appear against the backdrop of LNT premises) and the difficulties they face in being judged germane to policy development, consider the following question. If and when, through further testing, human cloning becomes technically feasible without the risk of undue physical harm to resulting offspring, would cloning be de-feasible as an option for couples—or even individuals—without some larger context for reflection than that of reproductive autonomy?

The attempt to identify what values might trump, or at least limit, the usual priority accorded individual reproductive rights, at its core raises questions about the adequacy of the LNT. Given constraints of space, I will not attempt here a frontal assault on that framework in systematic terms. Rather, I will develop several more modest points about the quality of our public discourse by using human cloning as a springboard for broader musings. It is quite instructive in debates on human cloning (and on many other issues in bioethics) to look closely at how we engage in public discussion and debate, for the conclusions we tend to reach, at the level of public policy, reveal several important aspects of our public conversation and of the way that we frame debates on contentious issues. First, as a matter of moral *method,* characteristic differences in conclusions drawn about the perils and prospects of cloning reflect different ways of "doing public morality," or thinking morally about public questions. Second, in considering the nature and scope of public moral reasoning, it is important to acknowledge the multifaceted character of our conversation and to appreciate that nearly all of us function in our deliberations as members of several "publics." Third, as members of various communities of discourse, we need not settle for the artificial constraints placed upon us by workaday distinctions between "public" and "private" morality. Virtually all of us "wear several hats" simultaneously, and a key challenge to our role as citizens is to make sense of these disparate claims upon our allegiance. A more robust vision of citizenship and of public reasoning, rather than restricting the range of our concern, can help us to understand the various *levels* of moral discourse available to us, the various *publics* to whom concerns are addressed, the different *contexts* within which various forms of arguments and appeals will have characteristic salience, and the various *forms of authority* appropriate to those different forms and levels of moral and political reflection.

Public Reasons and Public Reasoning

When discussing the appropriate basis for public policy, it is important to distinguish the justification of particular *acts* from the justification of social *practices.* This distinction, long familiar to readers of political theory, is especially pertinent to an issue such as human cloning. On the one hand, as noted above, opponents of cloning have offered various sorts of arguments. For some, especially within certain religious communities, there are deontological constraints on cloning based on the nature of sexuality itself or the meaning of procreation (although such positions might well be buttressed by other appeals).[14] For other opponents, the "larger" negative implications of allowing the prospect of human cloning are the primary basis of their concerns—an appeal to harmful consequences over time, rather than an objection based on the *intrinsic* nature of the act of cloning itself.

By contrast, for proponents of cloning, as evidenced in the testimony before NBAC, what seemed at work is largely an appeal to individual choices about reproduction. Within the current legally established framework of procreative rights, cloning, when determined to be biologically safe for the cloned individual, would emerge as simply one more option on the menu of reproductive choices.[15] Quite interestingly, however, proponents of cloning, rather than celebrating the general merits of cloning as a reproductive option, tend to appeal to "hard cases," often involving infertile couples, to make the "larger" case. Here a central irony emerges. Despite the maxim that "hard cases make bad law," proponents of human cloning usually appeal to a few emotionally laden cases to argue for a broad social policy supportive of cloning. Thus, they appeal to problematic individual cases to advance the case for unfettered personal choice. Moreover, the individual case, positively construed, is meant to be decisive for policy considerations in a way that the individual case, if construed in negative terms by opponents, is not. That asymmetry is prima facie surprising; one might have assumed that an appeal to individual cases would not be decisive for policy deliberations in either instance.

Unless, of course, something else is at stake. And surely, something else is at stake, at least as proponents of cloning develop their case. For central to the *moral* support for the prospect of human cloning is a primary appeal to the *legal* framework already in place regarding the legitimacy of putatively private reproductive choices. Notice that the focus has been restricted to a moral minimalism that allows primarily legal determinations to be morally decisive, apparently without remainder, from a policy perspective. Once a legal framework of rights is instantiated, all other appeals—emotional, moral, aesthetic, or religious—are relegated to a different, decidedly less influential level of discourse. Even when such appeals are deemed legitimate, they cannot, it appears, function as values to counter a currently protected "right" based on the satisfaction of reproductive desires.

What emerges, then, is not simply the distinction between individual acts and social practices and the different justifications required. For the focus on individual acts can lead to very different conclusions about their legitimacy, depending on whether one invokes deontological limits to morally licit human intervention or one appeals, consequentially, to the deleterious effects for some individuals in emotionally laden hard cases. What will be decisive in policy terms will be our judgments about the weight to be accorded such *individual* appeals in relation to larger *societal* concerns, which, according to the NBAC report, include the following: "[questions about] individuality, family integrity, and treating children as objects."[16]

Of course, the difficulty posed here is that we assume, with each new development, the trumping force of legal precedents in considering new possibilities that involve *both* legal and moral values. Granted, there are moral dimensions to the ascription of reproductive rights to individuals. But the status of a legal precedent in one instance (e.g., access to artificial insemination by donor or in vitro fertilization) may not, of itself, be dispositive of the *moral* dimensions of the current debate on human cloning. Stated most broadly, at issue is the tension posed for the theory of a liberal polity when differentiating the reasons that may justify a given act from those that should be decisive in justifying a social policy.

Communitarian Sources for Further Reflection

The challenges posed by new reproductive technologies and practices, including the prospect of human cloning, are profound. Given the silence of the LNT concerning the nature and scope of harms and benefits to children—beyond a minimal notion of the risk of physical harm—it is not surprising that the secular and religious critics of human cloning must look elsewhere in political and social theory to find the intellectual resources to accommodate their concerns. Communitarian thought has, in the last decade, criticized the moral minimalism that it sees at work in much of recent liberal theory on two basic grounds. First, the "denuded self" at the heart of recent social-contract theory fails to depict the more robust features of individuals as moral agents necessarily in community.[17] Second, communitarian thought criticizes the LNT for its failure to describe the full scope of our moral obligations, both as human beings and as citizens. Indeed, because not all—not even most—of our obligations are of the contractual variety, liberal political theory has, in recent years, had difficulty in accounting for the sense of "natural" duties that are central features of moral life and experience. Communitarianism incorporates such duties by distinguishing between autonomy as an abstract ideal and the conditions of what might be called "effective autonomy." Thus, communitarianism distinguishes itself sharply from libertarian thought by emphasizing positive rights as well as negative or noninterference rights. Effective autonomy, compared with autonomy in the abstract, will require certain communal conditions for the development and expression of individual autonomy. Specifically, with regard to the interests of children, communitarian thought might engage (though it largely has not) the sense of collective unease at work in many criticisms of the prospect of human cloning. For in communitarian thought, neither the language of individualism nor the call for social order assumes theoretical priority. Recent communitarian writings are extensive, and I cannot do them justice here. Instead, I will adduce several themes developed by Charles Taylor and Amitai Etzioni to indicate certain communitarian emphases that provide a corrective to the truncated view of self and society prevalent in recent liberal theory.

Among recent theorists, Charles Taylor has provided the most coherent philosophical description of our development as moderners. In his discussion, Taylor brilliantly describes one important strand of the modernist moral and political temper, which he describes as the "naturalist consciousness." This perspective, inspired by the instrumental success of natural science, distrusts alternative, apparently unresolvable, accounts of the good life and of what Taylor dubs the "ontology of the human."[18]

Although Taylor does not draw explicit parallels with the tenets of the LNT as a political paradigm, the implications of the naturalist consciousness in moral and political life are straightforward:

1. Because accounts of appropriate human ends apparently vary widely, political life and public policy formation should emphasize principles of the "right" (such as that of universal and equal respect) rather than notions of the good (including particular understandings of what constitutes psychological benefit or harm to children or appropriate notions of parenting).

2. Because notions of the substantive good vary widely, different accounts—beyond minimal standards of, say, preventing physical harm—are deemed incommensurable and therefore unavailable as the basis for restricting the rights of consenting adults in pursuit of their projects (including the project of parenting).

3. Insofar as a natural-science model has increasingly developed "on the basis of a conception of the world which is maximally freed from anthropocentric conceptions," what we call the "good" and the "right" are not deemed part of the "natural world."[19] They are either nonnatural, or projections, or simply human reactions of approval or disapproval relative to the visions and virtues defined by particular communities. Again, given the relativism among both individuals and communities, a public policy posture of agnosticism toward competing claims of the good emerges as the preferred strategy of accommodation. Particular perspectives as incommensurable are incapable of providing the shared

normative warrants sufficient to ground restrictive policy—
except for a "thin" understanding of harm, noncontroversially
shared, as the basis for social agreement.

In light of these implications of the "naturalist consciousness," it is
not surprising that the vision of moral agency at work in the LNT is
that of the "unencumbered" or "evacuated" self, a self devoid of shared
values of citizenship that could situate it decisively in community with
other selves in liberal society. The Rawlsian priority of the right, therefore, accords primacy of place to individual rights; the exercise of
human will, rather than a shared vision of the good, emerges as the
central emphasis of the LNT.

Apropos the case of human cloning, LNT principles play out to the
following conclusion. At some point, when issues of the physical safety
of the cloned child are addressed, the priority of the right over the
good will direct future policy. At that time, *because* reproductive rights
are the established legal context for considering parental choices, and
because individuals differ about the advisability of cloning as an option,
a public policy respectful of legal rights must accommodate those wishes.

The logic of Taylor's critique of naturalist consciousness (and, by
extension, the LNT) is complex. However, two points are especially
important to the richer mapping of the moral terrain required to critique
LNT premises. First, while Taylor acknowledges that the "good and
right are not part of the world as studied by natural science,"[20] he argues
that, in our capacity as moral agents, we *cannot* dispense with them,
as a matter of personal or political morality. The implication of Taylor's
linking of the good with the right makes the priority of the latter
untenable as a depiction of the ways that we actually engage in moral
reflection and deliberation. Taylor stresses what I deem an incontrovert-
ible point in this regard:

> What better measure of reality do we have in human affairs than those
> terms which on critical reflection and after correction of the errors we
> can detect make the best sense of our lives? "Making the best sense" here
> includes not only offering the best, most realistic orientation about the
> good but also allowing us best to understand and make sense of the actions
> and feelings of ourselves and others. For our language is continuous with
> our language of assessment, and this with the language in which we explain
> what people do and feel.[21]

Taylor makes a second point about the necessary linkage between
notions of the right and the good—that "[y]ou cannot help having

recourse to these strongly valued goods for the purposes of life: deliberating, judging situations, deciding how you feel about people, and the like."[22] Taylor does not view that linkage as univocal or necessarily determinative, for he acknowledges that individual and communal values—on the nature of parenting and other matters—will vary, both within and across societies. Taylor's point is not a denial of diversity, but an affirmation of the need for a richer account of morality—both personal and public—to make sense of the way that we actually operate in the moral realm. Moreover, on Taylor's account, the denuded self central to the LNT *must* be inadequate, even as a construct, because it fails to capture the intrinsic sense of *why* we value the right, the good, or the self who considers either of them, in the first place.

At the same time, Taylor is quite critical of monistic efforts, either Kantian or utilitarian, that seek to systematize our moral ends and obligations according to some "single reason," be it an assertion of the categorical imperative or a principle of utility.[23] Instead, Taylor celebrates the merits of a pluralistic account, in the lineage of Aristotle. Pluralism recognizes a number of basic goods as legitimate forms of human flourishing. It appreciates the need for our conduct, in pursuit of those ends, to exhibit virtues. Moreover, given the plurality of goods to be pursued, pluralism affirms the centrality of practical reason, which Taylor describes as "a reasoning in transitions," aiming to "establish not that some position is correct absolutely, but rather that some position is superior to some other."[24]

Taylor's affirmation of practical reason has two implications that bear critically on the premises of the LNT. First, because a "good life" may involve the pursuit of various goods, morality necessarily involves "articulating a vision" rather than simply "offering a reason." Taylor makes that subtle point in this way:

> . . . [A]rticulating a vision of the good is not offering a basic reason. It is one thing to say that I ought to refrain from manipulating your emotions or threatening you, because that is what respecting your rights as a human being requires. It is quite another to set out just what makes human beings worthy of commanding our respect, and to describe the higher mode of life and feeling which is involved in recognizing this. It is true that clarification on the second is closely related to the definition of the basic reasons we invoke in the first kind of claim. Our conceptions of what makes humans worthy of respect have shaped the actual schedule of rights we recognize, and the latter has evolved over the centuries with changes in the former. But they are nonetheless distinct activities.[25]

Second, the connection between a pluralistic axiology and the functioning of practical reason allows for, indeed, encourages, a moral discourse—in both the "internal" and the public forum—that will be attentive to the complexity of our deliberations; the indispensability of our intuitions; the "thick" accounts that we must provide to make sense of the world and of ourselves; and the various forms of argument, levels of authority, and appropriate forms of approbation and sanction we should pursue in both our personal and public projects. And while there is nothing in Taylor's general discussion that leads to specific policy conclusions—on human cloning or other issues—there is a great deal in his analysis that can be used to critique the LNT as a reliable or accurate description of, much less prescription for, either private or social morality.

Let me turn briefly to certain recent writings of Amitai Etzioni, perhaps the best-known expositor of communitarian thought. There are two core concepts to Etzioni's vision, all with implications for the way that we frame the cloning debate. First, in contrast to contractarian understandings, in a communitarian society, "*[V]alues are handed down from generation to generation rather than invented or negotiated*" (emphasis in the original).[26] This contrast between liberal individualism and communitarian thought is especially pronounced when questions about the interests of children are at issue. Etzioni emphasizes the contrast in these terms:

> The individualists' notion that social order will be negotiated or arranged . . . ignores the role of shared values . . . when the main beneficiaries are future generations. Children pose problems for libertarian theorists, who either assume children to be small individuals with the same rights as others or, much more commonly, ignore them. Obviously, neither future generations nor young children can be at the negotiation table to argue for their interests and conceptions of the good; instead, children are protected by our shared moral commitments that encompass them.[27]

A second core theme for Etzioni, which sharply distinguishes communitarian thinking from that of social conservative paradigms, involves his understanding of the appropriate relations that should obtain between social values and their expression in the law. In his words, "While communitarians basically have faith in and seek to convince people of the value of their position, relying on the moral voice of the community, education, persuasion, and exhortation, social conservatives are much more inclined to rely on the law to promote values in which they believe."[28] For Etzioni, it is crucially important to understand the core values that society does share, and that serve as the background features to many policy discussions. Thus, communitarian thinking emphasizes the need for both autonomy and social order and views the relationship between individual liberty and the common good in dialectical, rather than oppositional, terms. According to Etzioni, "for a society to be communitarian, much of the social conduct must be 'regulated' by reliance on the moral voice rather than on the law, and *the scope of the law itself must be limited largely to that which is supported by the moral voice*" (emphasis in the original).[29]

While I cannot speak with confidence about the concrete implications of Etzioni's writings for judgments about particular new reproductive technologies and practices (including the prospect of human cloning), his recommendations about how policy discussion should proceed reveal a vision that is far more robust than that of the LNT in several ways. First, there will be a "conservative" cast to the way that alternative arrangements in baby-making and child-rearing are assessed, by virtue of the equal importance that communitarian thought places on both the exercise of individual autonomy and the necessary social context for its effective development and emergence. Neither claims of reproductive freedom nor claims for uniquely normative patterns of parenting and family life will necessarily triumph. Instead, the core values upon which appropriate public policy is based will be clarified by a spirited public discussion and debate of alternative viewpoints. Second, Etzioni, in contrast to many of his critics, is confident about the possibility of extended moral dialogues, what he calls "megalogues," even in large-scale modern societies: "I argue that *whole societies, even a society whose population counts in the hundred of millions, do engage in moral dialogues* that lead to changes in . . . widely shared values. This process occurs by linking millions of local conversations . . . into society-wide networks and shared public focal points" (emphasis in the original).[30]

Finally, Etzioni speaks unabashedly about the various forms of suasion and moral authority at work in the broader communitarian conversation. In this respect, Etzioni's position differs noticeably from most versions of the LNT. As Etzioni notes, the LNT, drawing on the legacy of John Stuart Mill, usually finds "no principled difference between the coercion of the law and the urging of the moral voice."[31] By contrast, Etzioni supports extra-legal sanctions, especially societal attitudes of approbation and disapprobation, that, over time, may appropriately provide the shared basis for changing public policy, depending on the outcomes of ongoing "megalogues."

Cloning as a Methodological Prism: Toward a More Robust Policy Discussion

The debate about the prospect of human cloning is perhaps most instructive for what it reveals about deeper tendencies in our culture that I find quite troubling—the paucity of our moral categories, the poverty of our present moral discourse, and our seeming unwillingness or inability to reclaim or renew a language of the common good as a counterweight to that of personal autonomy and individual rights so prevalent in our society.

In 1984, Daniel Callahan spoke regretfully about the "moral minimalism" at work in the way we currently frame most public issues.[32] Indeed, Callahan's prescient phrase remains an apt description of recent policy discussion in bioethics. For many bioethicists, analytic philosophy is the *lingua franca* of ethical and policy discourse. Without shared reasons that can be clearly and compellingly articulated, we lack, apparently, any coherent basis for limiting individual action and choice. In making such requisite arguments, one must be logically compelling, systematic rather than merely suggestive, apodictical rather than allusive. Indeed, it would seem, one must dismiss all appeals to human imagination, human experience, and human intuition as too variable to be trustworthy as moral influences, much less as guides.

The prospect of human cloning, however, exemplifies the need for more than semantic coherence or rigorous argument in our moral musings and method about appropriate public policy. The assessment of cloning requires of us habits of the heart as well as of the mind. It requires of us the power of discernment, a way to "see through" things. In effect, we must be willing to view cloning as a prism, *through* which deeper themes and trends are refracted.

The various perspectives reviewed in the NBAC report reveal basic differences in both moral method and moral imagination. Note what is held, even if at times only subliminally, by proponents and opponents. On one side stand those who would appeal to human mastery, to technique, to new ways of responding to human misery—invariably, the examples used to carry the argument are sad individual cases. How dare we argue against the imperative of science, expressed in Francis

Bacon's dictum as "the relief of the human estate"? Who, save the inveterate pessimist, cannot find in the prospect of human cloning the possibility for some potential benefit in an individual case?

From the other side come a litany of objections—both religious and secular—some of which I have rehearsed. These critics, while not unsympathetic to the sadness of infertility or the desirability of overcoming genetic disease, embrace a fundamentally different, and I would suggest, broader, vantage from which to consider whether cloning offers greater peril or promise. Theirs is a worldview not reducible to clever argument; some matters of deep human import are too profound merely to be clever about. Theirs, instead, is a perspective that asks us to take seriously our own feelings and intuitions about ourselves, our attitudes about good parenting, and our awareness of the difference between seeing children as begotten or, increasingly, as products of our own specification. Theirs is a larger vision that asks us to look beyond particular cases, to set a wider aperture to our inquiry. In this method, to be accused of appealing to feeling, speculation, or imagination is not to suffer an insult, but to accept a compliment. From this perspective, what is most perilous about human cloning—beyond the issues I have already discussed—may be too deeply felt, too deeply human, and too important, to be reduced to rhetorical flourish or the tactics of debate.

In assessing the prospect of human cloning, and in reviewing the bases of both religious and secular arguments against it, certain common core values, when explored more fully and carefully than they have been to date, may well provide an effective counterweight to the excesses of liberal individualism. In exploring, albeit only in outline, the possibilities for convergence between religious and secular assessments, I have suggested that the "common ground" we find, while not perhaps fully articulable as a shared basis for pluralistic policy, remains relevant to the process of policy deliberation, and, of equal importance, to the way that policy choices will be *received* by the public.

If communitarianism is correct in its depiction of the relations between autonomy and community (and I believe that it is), we do well to celebrate the various facets of our public conversation and to reject the facile distinction between public and private morality that lies at the heart of the LNT. For in our moral, social, and political deliberations, virtually all of us, as citizens, are members of several "publics." We may be members of particular voluntary associations, including churches. We may serve as professional advisors or as members of appointed deliberative bodies, including ethics committees, institutional review boards, or advisory commissions. We may be appointed as representatives of particular constitutencies, with epistemologically privileged positions that we faithfully express in the larger public and policy conversation. The forms of authority that we invoke will vary, according to circumstances, as will the warrants, distinctive or shared, that we adduce to undergird our positions.

In different circumstances, we will employ different forms of moral discourse. As James Gustafson reminds us, such discourse, whether theologically inspired or not, functions in several ways. Gustafson discusses four types—what he calls ethical discourse, prophetic discourse, narrative discourse, and policy discourse. Each of them, he argues, is at some level necessary to the moral deliberations of particular communities and of society at large but none is, of itself, sufficient.[33] Of the four modes, we are probably most familiar with ethical discourse—the language of conseqentialism and deontology—and policy discourse—which works with the limited horizon of the values already embedded in our prior choices, and measures progress incrementally in the language of feasibility and compromise. Less familiar to our policy conversation, I fear, are the modes of prophecy and of narrative, the language of sweeping vision and of shaping stories. But the latter, I would suggest, are equally crucial to the public conversation about human cloning. For human cloning is not simply a matter of rights but also of responsibilities, not simply a question of reproductive liberties but also of parental duties, not merely a matter of new technical possibilities but of the ways that such possibilities enhance or diminish human freedom as a socially embedded reality.

In all of this, there are few easy answers. No single mode of discourse will suffice. But the premises of the LNT, as important as they may be procedurally, cannot be the last word on the character of our social conversation, on human cloning, or on any number of other contested issues. In this light, communitarian theory clearly supplies a necessary corrective to the moral minimalism we too often seem to settle for. We need the robustness of all voices being spoken and heard. We should not seek premature closure to a spirited, ongoing, and often frustrating public conversation. Indeed, the many levels of that conversation—its multidimensionality—rather than being a cause for consternation, can help to enrich the quality of our public discourse and correct the minimalism associated with the LNT. While it is true that law is sometimes conflated with morality, a subtler understanding of public discourse will not make that conceptual and practical mistake. Rather, the efforts—

by *both* speakers and hearers—to "translate" epistemologically privileged insights may result in a far richer conversation that can appeal beyond the blunt hand of law and regulation to other forms of moral and political suasion. And finally, even if, at some point, given precedents already established, we deem human cloning to be legally protected, we need not confuse that narrower judgment with broader moral or societal approval.

NOTES

1. Bruce Ackerman, "Why Dialogue?" *Journal of Philosophy* 86, no. 1 (1989): 5–22, at 16: "When you and I learn that we disagree about one or another dimension of the moral truth, we should not search for some common value that will trump this disagreement; nor should we try to translate it into some putatively neutral framework; nor should we seek to transcend it by talking about how some unearthly creature might resolve it. We should simply say *nothing at all* about this disagreement and put the moral ideals that divide us off the conversational agenda of the liberal state."

2. Gilbert C. Meilaender, testimony before the National Bioethics Advisory Commission, 13 March 1997.

3. For a recent exposition of Rawls's thought on the functioning of "public reason," see John Rawls, "The Idea of Public Reason Revisited," *University of Chicago Law Review* 64, no. 3 (1997): 765–807.

4. The National Bioethics Advisory Commission (hereinafter NBAC), *Cloning Human Beings: Report and Recommendations of the National Bioethics Advisory Commission* (Rockville, Md.: June 1997), pp. 3, 34, 107–110.

5. Leon Kass, "The Wisdom of Repugnance," in Leon R. Kass and James Q. Wilson, *The Ethics of Human Cloning* (Washington, D.C.: AEI Press, 1998), pp. 3–59.

6. NBAC, *Cloning Human Beings*, pp. 39–61.

7. Nancy Duff, testimony before the National Bioethics Advisory Commission, 13 March 1997.

8. NBAC, *Cloning Human Beings*, p. 56.

9. Kass, "The Wisdom of Repugnance," pp. 3–59.

10. Philip Boyle, comments as a member of The Hastings Center Working Group on Biotechnology and Religion, April 1997.

11. Oliver O'Donovan, *Begotten or Made?* (Oxford: Clarendon Press, 1984), p. 16.

12. Kass, "The Wisdom of Repugnance," p. 38.

13. Allen Verhey, "Theology After Dolly," *Christian Century* (March 19–26, 1997): 285–86, at 285.

14. Albert S. Moraczewski, testimony before the National Bioethics Advisory Commission, 13 March 1997.

15. John A. Robertson, testimony before the National Bioethics Advisory Commission, 14 March 1997.

16. NBAC, *Cloning Human Beings*, p. ii.

17. Michael J. Sandel, "Justice and the Good," in *Liberalism and Its Critics*, ed. Michael J. Sandel (New York: New York University Press, 1984), pp. 159–76.

18. Charles Taylor, *Sources of the Self* (Cambridge, Mass.: Harvard University Press, 1989), p. 5.

19. Taylor, *Sources of the Self*, p. 56.

20. Taylor, *Sources of the Self*, p. 56.

21. Taylor, *Sources of the Self*, p. 57.

22. Taylor, *Sources of the Self*, p. 57.

23. Taylor, *Sources of the Self*, p. 76.

24. Taylor, *Sources of the Self*, p. 72.

25. Taylor, *Sources of the Self*, p. 77.

26. Amitai Etzioni, *The New Golden Rule: Community and Morality in a Democratic Society* (New York: Basic Books, 1996), p. 93.

27. Etzioni, *The New Golden Rule*, p. 95.

28. Etzioni, *The New Golden Rule*, p. 16.

29. Etzioni, *The New Golden Rule*, p. 139.

30. Etzioni, *The New Golden Rule*, p. 106.

31. Etzioni, *The New Golden Rule*, p. 132.

32. Daniel Callahan, "Minimalist Ethics," *Hastings Center Report* 11, no. 5 (1981): 19–25.

33. James Gustafson, "Moral Discourse About Medicine: A Variety of Forms," *Journal of Medicine and Philosophy* 15, no. 2 (1990): 125–42.

John H. Evans

The Uneven Playing Field of the Dialogue on Patenting[1]

I have sensed that the public dialogue about patenting DNA has been subtly biased. Although dialogue implies a two-way examination, it has seemed that the debate has only been an interrogation of the ideas and arguments of the religious groups that have raised concerns about patenting. In the dialogue that I have been a part of,[2] participants have focused on what religious advocates "really" mean by their statements; or to take a more precise example, what "really" concerns them about "commodification." I have not witnessed an equivalent plumb of arguments of the other side of the dialogue, the proponents of patenting. Biotechnology companies seem to proceed as if their arguments were somehow neutral, obvious, or not requiring scrutiny, thereby placing the burden of proof on the religious leaders to defend the logic of their arguments.

The operating assumption seems to be that the biotechnology industry is innocent until proven guilty and the opponents are guilty until proven innocent. For example, reacting to the press conference of the Coalition Against Patenting, Biotechnology Industry Organization president, Carl Feldbaum, dismisses the coalition's actions as "misinformed," but "sincere." He concludes that in the view of his organization, "no one can or should own life itself."[3] This is an equally cryptic claim as any spoken by the religious groups. What does the phrase "to own" mean if not a patent?[4] More important, what is "life itself" and how is this different from what opponents mean by "life"? Why is it that the claims of the religious opponents demand scrutiny and the equally cryptic claims of the biotechnology industry do not? It seems to me that claims of both sides in a dialogue require equal scrutiny. However, the fact that the debates have not done so demonstrates to me that the playing field has been tilted against the religious opponents of patenting.

A Dialogue to Strive For

Perhaps the problem is that the two sides have different reasons for being at the same table. One gets the sense that dialogue for industry is actually public relations, because the representatives are structurally constrained by their employment so that they could not agree with the opponents of patenting. I will assume in this chapter that both sides intend to have a particular form of dialogue: They intend to strive to truly understand each other in search of a consensus on a course of action. This might also be called dialogue in good faith. I assume that the point of dialogue is also *not* information gathering about your opponents so as to be able to make more effective counterarguments. This would be called something like politics. Striving for a consensus is a process that of course may or may not lead to a consensus as the outcome. I focus here on the process, not the substance or outcome of the dialogue. Nor, should I add, do I want to be taken as saying that one "side" is right or wrong in its conclusions.

There are a number of conditions that must be satisfied for unbiased dialogue to occur. I will focus on one condition, that the striving for consensus and dialogue implies that the players have equal standing at the table—that the table is not tilted in one direction—and that any outcome can occur.[5] Although there is a voluminous literature on this topic,[6] I will focus on only one precondition for this equal standing: that the standards used to determine what a good argument is are shared by all participants. I will ignore all of the other preconditions that may or may not be satisfied for dialogue—unequal power or information of the participants, charisma, small group dynamics, and the like.

Standards of Evaluation in the Patenting Dialogue

What is a "good argument" about patenting? Not surprisingly, people of goodwill disagree. It is also commonplace to assume that the assumptions people bring to the table affect this evaluation. A useful theoretical metaphor for these assumptions is the idea of a "frame," which Erving Goffman thought of as a "schemata of interpretation" that allows people to "locate, perceive, identify and label" occurrences within the world.[7] The insight here is that we cannot simply absorb all of the phenomena that occur before us during the day, but must be able to categorize them to help us in analysis. If every event occurred de novo, we would be overwhelmed by the task of going through every possible meaning of the event in our heads, essentially reinventing the wheel at every moment.

Issue Frames

When people hear of a new issue that they do not understand, they also try to put it into a schema of interpretation or frame that they already have at hand in order to be able to understand it. This is one reason why the abortion debate seems to seep into other issues. As the most readily available frame for understanding the political aspects of reproduction, new reproductive technology questions often are "framed" using the frame of the abortion debate, with its prepackaged cognitive categories (e.g., conflict of rights among different forms of life) that may or may not be the best way to consider the new issue. The debate then focuses on the parts of the phenomenon for which there are categories (e.g., conflicts over rights), while ignoring other parts of the phenomenon.

This sociological insight is not lost on policy advocates who learn to "define the terms of the debate" and "set the agenda." I will cast this as the *issue frame*, and organizations spend millions of dollars trying to influence this in the public mind. For example, is nicotine an addictive drug? There is no objective definition of addiction, but there are great interests at stake in trying to make sure it is framed as a lifestyle choice, and thus placing it cognitively with what soda we drink, rather than placing it cognitively with heroin. It is the issue frame that determines who legitimately makes the decisions. If nicotine is a drug, cigarettes become a policy issue decided by legislatures, the courts, and executive branch agencies. If it is a lifestyle choice, the decisions remain with individuals.

If the debate is defined as about "patenting," then a particular set of arguments will be what is immediately accessed in our minds. A patent is a legal construction about property, and items defined as being about "patenting" will seem more "naturally" to be amenable to forms of argumentation that are used with law, property, and public policy. Moreover, what to do about "patenting" will more likely be decided in the institutions of government that usually concern themselves with these issues.

However, this is not the only way that we could *frame* the *issue*. A reading of some of the religious leaders' statements who oppose patenting of DNA suggests that the issue being debated might just as easily be framed as something like a "meaning-of-life" *issue frame*. Bishop

Kenneth Carder of the United Methodist Church said at a press conference announcing a coalition to stop patenting that the debate is actually about "the commodification of life and the reduction of life to its commercial value."[8] From this *issue frame*, the debate should not be about patenting; patenting is only one symptom of the actual problem. If the issue was initially framed in this manner, a reasonable dialogue might not include legal, scientific, and policy specialists because they have limited expertise in defining what the commodification of life is. Instead, decisions about the commodification of life might be decided by individuals, religious institutions, or families, and government institutions would be less likely to be involved.

It seems indisputable that this dialogue has been framed as being about patent policy—the titles given to the dialogues are evidentiary. I suspect that the religious groups would rather not be arguing about patents, but rather about the commodification of life. But, for reasons too complex to enter into here, the mainline religions that initiated this effort tend to not be able to successfully frame the issues, but rather tend to be reactive. The point is that by having the debate *defined as being* about patenting, instead of the broader issue of commodification with patenting DNA as a symptom, the religious groups are already arguing about a side argument to their actual stated concerns. This is the first slant in the playing field.

Argumentative Frames

Just as issues are framed, the types of arguments that we make are embedded in frames that I will call *argumentative frames*. These are, once again, the assumptions or preconceived cognitive categories that highlight what part of the phenomenon is important. They include assumptions about the grounds for evaluating arguments as legitimate or illegitimate. Below I juxtapose two ideal-type *argumentative frames* that I believe are represented in this dialogue. These categories—an amalgam of the theories of James Gustafson, Daniel Callahan, and Jeffrey Stout[9]—are the "ethical" and the "prophetic."[10]

As a general orientation, claims in the ethical frame are micro-level, while claims in the prophetic frame are macro-level. While in the ethical frame the point is to try to figure out what one is supposed to do in particular circumstances, in the prophetic frame the claimant is typically not occupied with the surface issues but is rather concerned with exposing the roots of what is perceived to be fundamentally and systematically right or wrong. In Gustafson's words, "prophets are seldom interested in specific acts except insofar as they signify a larger and deeper evil or danger."[11]

In the ethical frame, the actor who is the concern of the claim and the one who should act is the individual. In the prophetic frame, the actor in question is often the entirety of humanity. Ethical arguments focus on concrete acts that are clearly immediate and future questions are put off until they become immediate, while a prophetic analysis peers into the future. The prophetic frame uses a vision of what the good life is, as well as what the wider and deeper consequences of incremental developments are.

In its mode of reasoning, the ethical frame uses the application of principles to cases and the sharpening of distinctions between cases. Arguments using the prophetic frame often question the very principles that are used in ethical discourse. Subjective claims such as emotion and perception are bracketed as either unimportant or unusable in the ethical frame. The prophetic, on the other hand, often considers emotional responses to be signals of wisdom. In argumentation, therefore, the prophetic often uses appeals to affect rather than to reason.

Public Policy Issue Framing and the Associated Argumentative Frame

I will now turn to how framing an issue regarding public policy, and patent policy in particular, tilts the playing field against the prophetic argumentative frame. The basic point here is that government institutions tend to have frames institutionalized into their decision-making processes as well, and these frames are generally of the ethical variety. I will elaborate on two of these constraints on government that result in the bias toward the ethical frame and the bias against the prophetic frame.

Government Action as "Visible"

As pointed out by political scientist Yaron Ezrahi, government action has to be observable to be legitimate.[12] For example, government officials cannot simply "believe" that gene patenting is wrong; they have to "show" or, better yet, "prove" with scientific methods, that gene patenting is wrong in order to restrict it. This may seem obvious because we are so used to expecting this from our representatives. However, this is an important distinction because it means that if your argument depends on claims that are not "demonstrable" or, in a stronger version, "provable" using science, it is not a legitimate argument. I will merely point out here—and elaborate on below—the fact that not only do the theological claims of religious groups ("God owns life") fall short of this standard, but so do their secular claims ("patenting is commodification").

This first form of constraint on arguments used in policy claims is one of the factors that leads to the dominance of cost-benefit analysis in public policy. Cost-benefit analysis and other consequentialist forms of reasoning purport to "show" the public the legislative process. If the costs and benefits cannot be shown, it is unclear how decisions should be made given the need to prove what will happen with policy. If it can't be shown, it is illegitimate because it might not be benefiting the entire society but actually only an influential subgroup.

I will use data from the process whereby the President's Commission for Study of Ethical Problems in Medicine and Biomedical and Behavioral Research of the early 1980s created the report on human genetic engineering titled *Splicing Life*[13] as examples of these constraints and the effect of these constraints on argumentative frames.[14] The first example is of an argument that is incompatible with the constraint that public policy claims have to be able to show their effects.

Leon Kass of the University of Chicago makes a number of arguments using a prophetic argumentative frame during the President's Commission process. His primary criticism was that the commission's form of analysis is to begin with what is technically possible and then decide what the society should do. He argues that the commission should start with human values and derive what should be technologically accomplished to satisfy these values. He also reacts to an argument that emotional responses should be ignored by questioning the very basis of this response: "The concerns expressed in such phrases as 'playing God' or 'dehumanization' are expressions of wisdom, even if passionately expressed and poorly argued for. What my fellow scientists call 'emotional' may be more *reasonable* than the *rational*, coldly 'objective' opinions with which they contend."[15] Finally, in reaction to a view of a participant that the commission should only address issues that may occur in the immediate future because "future changes in the technology or in human values may alter the nature of the problem," he responded that the "things that are most significant are not close at hand."

These arguments fit well within the prophetic argumentative frame. Debate is about human values, not human genetic engineering. Kass considers human genetic engineering a surface issue for the deeper question of values. His analysis peers into the future and has a vision of what the good life is. The actor in question is humanity (human values), not the potential individual recipient of the technology.

These arguments had little influence on the proceedings, not because they were poorly made, but rather because they originate from an argumentative frame that is incompatible with the state (government) constraints. My interpretation of the process whereby the commission rejected Kass's arguments is that they were rejected because the costs and benefits of his claims could not be calculated into the murky future; thus, "provable," "demonstrable" action required in the state context is not possible. "Playing God," as a claim of cost or harm, is not measurable because it cannot be defined in the same currency as the benefit—the amelioration of disease and human suffering.[16] Moreover, potential acts in the distant future cannot have costs and benefits assigned to them because, as one commissioner noted, our "human values" may change and we might place a different price on different actions. This is an example of how politics as an "observable, factual reality" has an "implicit commitment to the normative superiority of the present over the past and the future."[17]

Kass's concerns were eventually bracketed as interesting, but not something the commission should deal with. It was concluded that the government should consider these problems later, when they became more imminent. If we reflect on this a moment, we can see that addressing Kass's concerns in the future is equivalent to not addressing them, because concerns about the future must be addressed before the future arrives. The constraint of demonstrable effects and costs thus subtly works against prophetic arguments.

I digress to simply note that the employees of the commission and the commissioners are not deceitful or vicious people. Commissioners wanted to have a report that would be accepted and useful. From the standards needed to have an accepted and useful report in the context, Kass makes no sense. Therefore, my point is not about the maliciousness of persons in either the President's Commission or the dialogue on patenting, but rather that constraints outside the control of any of the individuals involved with the commission and the dialogue resulted in the marginalization of a certain type of claim.

The Removal of Nuance in State Decision Making

The second constraint on making claims to the state that I will raise may also seem obvious but once again is important. In my earlier research on these forms of argumentation in the debate about human genetic engineering from the 1950s to the present, I made a subtle finding that I did not make much of at the time. The prophetic framed arguments were longer—much longer. The prophetic voices generally required entire books to make their arguments, while the ethical claims could be made in short journal articles. Basically, prophetic arguments involve more information, and are subtler.

Many have noted that ethical decision-making processes preferred by the state such as risk-benefit and cost-benefit analysis are basically systems for throwing away information to make the decision-making process easier[18] and, in Ezrahi's terms, more "visible." This bias toward throwing away of information is evident in the patenting debate as well. To put it quite simply, participants in a debate *framed as being about public policy* are not encouraged to say "maybe."

You have to support a bill or oppose it. You sign the statement of the Coalition on Patenting or you don't. You make a statement or you don't. More important, after a threshold of "yes" is reached, you are in support; your processes, equivocations, and nuances to get to that point are generally ignored. And, since your nuances in this binary "yes/no" decision-making process are generally ignored, you are believed to be wholly in support of your past "yes" decisions—an unequivocal yes without the reality of the often equivocal yes. There is also a tendency to treat past political inaction for whatever reason as implicit support.

In American politics, you are expected to be consistent. If you sign one statement and not another, you are expected to come up with a principle of distinction between the two cases so that your beliefs can be further clarified. If you approve of patenting plants but not animals, then you must come up with a "principle of distinction" between the two cases or be held to be irrational according to the norms of the policy process.

Taking another example from the President's Commission, the impetus for the commission starting the study on human genetic engineering in the first place was the claim by religious leaders that changing the human genome is "playing God." The melding of state constraints and forms of argumentation is exemplified by the most prominent response in that commission to this "playing God" claim, which was, in the words of one commissioner, that scientists "have played God for quite some time." In fact, "the whole development of medicine . . . is in fact playing God, keeping people alive . . . who otherwise would have died."[19] This accepted medicine, in turn, affects the human genome through human intervention, not divine intervention.

The prophetic argument about playing God therefore is discredited as being senseless. In fact, it is, from within the constraints of the government commission and the ethical argumentative frame. It violates the constraint that "no maybe's" are allowed. This counterargument works because it appeals to the constraint that people who make claims in an issue framed as regarding public policy have to stand by fixed yes/no positions that they have previously explicitly advocated or implicitly advocated through previous inaction. Thus, this argument goes, you approve of medicine saving people who otherwise would have died ("yes"), and this changes the genome ("yes"), and you don't call medicine "playing God" ("yes"); thus, your "playing God" argument makes no sense.

However it is only senseless when evaluated from this perspective. In places where the prophetic argumentative frame is the standard of evaluation, the shades of gray that exist in everyone's position are allowed to be factored into the statement. Thus, evaluated from a prophetic frame, the first two steps of the argument remain the same: You approve of medicine saving people who otherwise would have died ("yes"), and this changes the genome ("yes"). In the final stage of this argument, if we allow ambiguity, the argument retains coherence. The actual nuance of the situation is that although users of the phrase "playing God" do not call medicine "playing God" and they acknowledge that medicine has some God-like qualities, that they wholeheartedly and unambiguously support medicine is a false assumption structured into the argument by the constraint of never being able to say "maybe." Allowing different degrees of "playing God" therefore results in a different evaluation of this argument.

The Argumentative Frames in the Patenting Debate

The implication of the above is that because the *issue* at hand is *framed* as about "patenting," rather than "commodification" or some other topic, it is being debated in a policy context. Furthermore, I have shown how the policy context selects against prophetic argumentative frames. I will use a few sample arguments from the dialogue on patenting genes to make the general claim that the religious opponents of patenting use the prophetic argumentative frame and the industry supporters of patenting use the ethical frame, and thus the table is tilted against the opponents.

Opponents of Patenting

According to Bishop Kenneth Carder of the United Methodist Church,[20] the concern with patenting DNA is "the commodification of life and the reduction of life to its commercial values and marketability." Note how hard participants in the dialogue have tried to understand this. What is commodification? How do we define it? Also note that, like Kass's comments, this claim is not measurable using cost-benefit analysis because the cost of the "commodification" of life is entirely unclear. This is because unlike the ethical frame, which has a common currency of demonstrable harms and benefits to individuals, the harmed entity is society, which cannot be readily compared to individuals.[21]

Take another argument of opponents: "God owns life and therefore no one should be able to patent an animal." Attempts at translation of this argument into arguments compatible with the ethical argumentative frame result in arguments easily discounted by these standards. Even when opponents try to put this in ethical terms, it does not make sense at the level of analysis.

The counterargument to this claim is typically: "Doesn't God own plants and you aren't opposed to patenting plants?" Evaluated from the standpoint of ethical frame, which makes the most sense in public policy claims, this is a devastating critique until someone can articulate a "principle" that separates plants from animals since God presumably owns both. The argument goes like this: (1) if you disapprove of patenting animals, you must logically (2) disapprove of patenting plants (because you can't come up with a principle of distinction between plants and animals) and (3) you are not opposed to patenting plants, so (4) your position is illogical.

But, from the prophetic frame, this is not much of a critique. As stated above, this form of counterargument assumes that people don't have more nuanced positions than the yes/no answers that "rational" policy processes force on them (approve or disapprove, sign the statement or not). However, if we accept nuance at every step, we will see that: (1) opponents disapprove of patenting animals; (2) they accept patenting of plants, but are actually ambivalent about it, because they are concerned about power and private ownership in general. The somewhat socialist strands of Methodist social teaching (and the entire Christian tradition) attest to this ambivalence. So, (3) although they are not opposed to patenting plants, their position (4) about patenting animals is not illogical, because they have always had a nuanced tension in their beliefs about private property and power of others, that just didn't quite hit the "oppose" threshold for plants. It is not difficult to imagine that had the political conditions been different at the historical point that patents were granted on plants, the Methodists would have opposed plant patenting.

Is this nuanced tension between principles illogical or improper? Whatever our evaluation of it, the Methodists to some extent have no choice if they want to remain Methodists. It has been said that the entire liberal Christian tradition is built upon "attempting to maintain the tensions" inherent in Christian theology.[22] From this perspective, each theological position or social concern is a virtue "only when held in tension with its counterpart."[23] This may account for the disinclination to define the stations of the continua that separate the ideas in tension. This feature of Methodist and other liberal Protestant theology might be a disadvantage if they were operating the U.S. courts, but may be considered less of a problem when discussing societal goals.

Proponents of Patenting

Proponents of patenting make counterarguments using entirely dif- ferent criteria, ethical arguments that more naturally align with what is expected when making public policy claims. Here I will use published arguments from George Poste of SmithKline Beecham Pharmaceuticals as an example. His counterargument against the prophetic arguments that are outside of the frame of patent law is that "it is neither appropriate nor productive to expect patent law to resolve issues it was never designed to address."[24] I have also heard this articulated as "you don't fight that fight at the patent office." Within the ethical frame—and highly consistent with modern policymaking—the focus is always on the micro-question at hand: patenting. Restricting analysis to the micro- question aids in making rational decisions.

Within the prophetic frame, the whole point is to fight the larger fight at the patent office, because the patent office is the symptom to which the prophet points to convince the people of the larger problem. In the Christian tradition this form or argument is ubiquitous. An ethical analysis of Jesus turning over the tables of the money changers in the temple would say that Jesus should not have picked on the money changers, but should have taken his complaints to the source, the society that allowed profiteering of the poor. In the prophetic tradition, attacking the money changers serves as a vehicle to take the complaints to the source.

Poste's main argument also uses an implicit cost-benefit analysis. He claims that the cost of banning DNA patenting is that pharmaceutical companies will not do the research to produce new drugs to improve human health: "Given that a patent is an essential prerequisite for commercial development of a gene into a medicine . . . denying the patentability of genes would mean that they would not be developed into innovative new products. This would betray the moral obligation to relieve suffering and would be deeply unethical."[25] He then shows how there are no benefits to banning DNA patents by saying "opponents of patents on DNA have yet to demonstrate a single case in which an individual or community has been damaged by the grant of a patent on DNA."[26] His conclusion is thus that "opponents claim that a patent on a DNA strand is unethical, but closer scrutiny reveals that the converse is true."[27]

Using the ethical frame, this argument wins out. The opponents of patenting cannot show a person who has been damaged by the grant of a patent. However, only in an ethical frame does this work. From a prophetic frame the benefits of banning patenting are not measurable on an individual level or probably even measurable at the standards required by policy analysis. In the prophetic frame you would not expect to find a person damaged by a patent to DNA in a concrete sense. Rather, prophets would claim that the individual is harmed in that the collective sense of human purpose is being damaged. Should this form of harm, albeit difficult to define, be excluded from dialogue?

The Problem of Translation

To sum up where I have gone so far, I am saying that the opponents of DNA patenting make arguments using a prophetic frame and that proponents of patenting use an ethical frame. My research shows that arguments using an ethical frame are more easily accepted as legitimate by state policymakers. The following objection could be raised: Religious advocates with prophetic frames or argumentation have always had to translate their claims in the public sphere, and this has worked well.

It is indisputable that prophets, particularly of the religious variety, have learned to be "bilingual," using the prophetic frame for their arguments at certain points and the ethical frame at others.[28] For example, a few paragraphs after the sentence I quoted from Bishop Carder about the commodification of life, he offers an implicit acceptance of the cost-benefit type of analysis. He offers an anticipatory response to Poste's claim that banning patents will stop research by saying that research had continued during a moratorium on patenting animals. Moreover, opponents of patenting come to the dialogue prepared to debate patent law. In fact, in my experience, the most successful denominational public policy advocates are those who are not only bilingual, but who can link the ethical arguments made in Congress to the prophetic arguments they make to motivate their own people in the pews.[29]

However, these ethical arguments always seem weak. That is because advocates really don't believe in them. They are just translating for the sake of participating in the policy process, that is, of being relevant in the debate. At the President's Commission, people who used prophetic arguments either had their arguments defeated, had to try to translate their arguments into arguments that were compatible with the constraints of the Presidential Commission, or had their arguments translated for them when they didn't do an effective enough job of providing alternative language. What really concerns opponents of patenting is, in my opinion, the prophetic arguments: After all, why would they utter them at all if they know they have little currency in policy debates?

The reason why this system does not work well is that it violates the terms of dialogue that I described above because the people who must translate have one hand tied behind their backs. To see the disadvantage, imagine a seminary that has just been purchased by a state university. The professors are told that they can still train future Christian pastors about the concepts of grace, atonement, and the trinity, but that they can only use a list of 10,000 words that were uttered in the physics building last month. Assuming that this was not finals time with undergraduate appeals for divine intervention in the exam process, these professors would have a very hard time. They could possibly do it, but I think they would have a harder time convincing the students that physicists could not answer these same questions more effectively. To sum up, your arguments lack power when translated into a second argumentative frame whose underlying logic you may understand but do not ultimately believe.

Suggestions for Heightened Dialogue

If we do want to make the dialogue more even, what can we do? I have a few tentative proposals for an improved dialogue that make it less structured against persons using the prophetic argumentative frame. The first is simply recognition from persons on both sides of the debate that their opponents are using different frames for their arguments. It has been argued that the standard move in *political* debate (rather than dialogue) is to try to demonstrate that your opponent is outside the bounds of the taken-for-granted principles of the nation, equivalent to demonstrating that someone is un-American.[30] In the patenting dialogue, this same political move occurs when the dialogue partner's arguments are shown to be outside the frame being used—as if the frame being used is the benchmark of reasonable argument. This is very effective for politics, but not conducive to taking your opponent's claims seriously in a dialogue.

I would propose a moratorium on claims that your opponent's arguments do not make sense using *your* preferred frame, as if they shared this frame. For example, Poste's claim that the opponents of patenting are wrong because they can't find someone hurt by patenting would violate this moratorium. This proposal would require persons in dialogue to learn each other's frames—like learning another language. At present, this would mostly fall on industry because religious advocates for public policy are already bilingual, even if they do not acknowledge it. As a very concrete suggestion, we should adopt the requirements of writing a book review for a journal. In a fair critique you are required to state your opponent's position so well that they agree with your rendering of it. For this dialogue, persons should be given an equally accurate description of the frame of argument that the position is based in, as well as an account of the argument itself. Poste would then have to include a sentence that said something like: "Opponents of patenting view harm as incurring on all of humanity, which cannot be readily compared to the benefits I describe above." Or, a parallel suggestion would be to acknowledge the other's frame and argue against the application of that frame to the issue at hand.

The tougher question is how to make the policy sphere less slanted against the prophetic claim. I still believe that people *should* be forced to translate explicitly transcendent prophetic claims into secular prophetic claims—I don't think that people should legitimately be able to say that "God commands this of us" when making laws. However, in the current situation, all prophetic claims, religious and secular, are eliminated from these debates. Religious prophetic claims can be translated into secular language. For example, at the President's Commission, Leon Kass's series of prophetic arguments were very similar to those expressed by others in explicitly theological language. This is the compromise that religious people will have to make.[31] In justification, I simply point to what I believe to be the success of the First Amendment to the Constitution for believer and nonbeliever alike.

But, how can even secular prophetic arguments become more accepted in public debates? That is, how do we lower the constraints I have observed? First, I would argue that ultimately the constraints I identified are based in the beliefs of policymakers and advocates of policy that if they do not adhere to them the government will not be legitimate in the eyes of its citizens. I believe that through making prophetic claims in the public arena and insisting on their legitimacy in the process, participants will find that the citizens are not as wedded to these constraints as they have supposed. For example, the citizenry accepts all sorts of goals of the government that cannot be proven. We accept that economic growth is good, we accept the idea that technological progress will make us happier, and we accept the idea that preservation of the family as the dominant social institution is best. These claims seem equally impervious to empirical factual argument as any of the prophetic claims described above.

The standard way of arguing against the prophetic within bioethics is to say that there is no societal consensus about prophetic claims, but that there is about the bases of ethical claims. Thus, the argument continues, to use "thick" notions of the good (part of the prophetic frame) in public policy would violate the deeply held beliefs of some part of the population and would thus be unjust. The "thin," ethical proceduralist wing of bioethics is well represented by the view that there are four "principles" of society that should be maximized: autonomy, beneficence, nonmaleficence, and justice. I suspect that this view is correct. If I created a public opinion poll, I would find that a strong majority of the public holds these as principles, and the conclusion would therefore be that they are justly applied to society.

I suspect that I could also find nearly equivalent support for a translated "prophetic principle" that "not everything in life should have a price." Certainly there is as much consensus over what that statement means as there is over the supposedly consensual principle of "justice." As I have written elsewhere, we often forget that the motivation for the creation of the bioethics "principles" was a request by Congress.[32] What we believe to be shared, pluralistic beliefs, may have been shaped by the tendency toward the ethical frame in government that I have noted above.

This suggests a bit more of a radical solution to the problem: democracy. I suspect that the prophetic frame has more of a following with U.S. citizens than with the U.S. elite. Note, for example, that the abortion debate is almost entirely prophetic on both sides, and the state, science, industry, and bioethics are relatively uninvolved.[33] As others have pointed out, science and industry are technocratic enterprises,[34] as is bioethics.[35] The educational process itself that makes people into members of the elite (us?) generally teaches a form of argumentation analogous to the focused frame. A good deal of the bias against the prophetic frame would therefore be alleviated if these dialogues involved a wider selection of the citizens of this country.

The proponents of patenting put forward an unequivocal good: the furthering of medical technologies for the relief of physical pain and suffering in our fellow humans. However, I would argue that other human values have long been a part of discussions of the public good. If the relief of physical pain and suffering of individuals is the only human value considered in a dialogue, this should be because it is agreed upon, not because it is a value expressed in a form of reasoning amenable to policy decisions. As pointed out by Gustafson, if the solution of a problem occurs solely within one of these frames and not another, then "significant issues of concern to morally sensitive persons and communities" will be left unattended.[36]

NOTES

1. This chapter is a revised version of an essay that was published in *Perspectives on Genetic Patenting: Religion, Science and Industry in Dialogue*, ed. Audrey R. Chapman (Washington, D.C.: American Association for the Advancement of Science, 1999), pp. 57–73. It is being used with the permission of the Program of Dialogue on Science, Ethics, and Religion of the American Association for the Advancement of Science. I am grateful to the participants at The Hastings Center meeting for their helpful criticism and to the American Association for the Advancement of Science for permission to revise and reprint this essay here.

2. I was a participant in a three-meeting dialogue on this topic at The Hastings Center from June 1996 to April 1997. I would also like to apologize for a certain bias of my own, which is that my discussion disproportionately focuses on liberal Protestant opponents at the expense of others due to their greater documentation on the topic as well as my greater familiarity both academically and personally with this community over others.

3. Reginald Rhein, "Gene Patent Crusade Moving from Church to Court," *Biotechnology Newswatch* (5 June 1995): 1.

4. I am aware that technically and legally a patent is not ownership. However, in common use of the term, patents give limited rights that most people would associate with ownership. Relying on a legal definition of "to own," while opponents use a more common understanding, is indicative of the problem I am concerned with.

5. Bruce Jennings, "Possibilities of Consensus: Toward Democratic Moral Discourse," *Journal of Medicine and Philosophy* 16, no. 4 (1991): 447–63, at 455.

6. Jonathan D. Moreno, *Deciding Together: Bioethics and Moral Consensus* (New York: Oxford University Press, 1995).

7. Erving Goffman, *Frame Analysis* (Cambridge, Mass.: Harvard University Press, 1974), p. 21.

8. Kenneth Carder, "A Statement on Patenting of Genes," Statement presented at the National Press Club, Washington, D.C., 18 May 1995.

9. James M. Gustafson, "Moral Discourse about Medicine: A Variety of Forms," *Journal of Medicine and Philosophy* 15 (1990): 125–142; Daniel Callahan, "Why America Accepted Bioethics," *Hastings Center Report*, November/December (1993): S8–S9; Jeffrey Stout, *Ethics After Babel* (Boston, Mass.: Beacon Press, 1988).

10. In religious communities this term is often associated with the condemnation of the majority of the people by the prophet, or with the prophet being instructed by God. In a modern, milder form, liberal church leaders taking positions more liberal than their members—and conservative church members taking positions more conservative than their members—often consider themselves "prophetic." These are not the senses in which I use the term.

11. Gustafson, "Moral Discourse about Medicine," p. 130.

12. Yaron Ezrahi, *The Descent of Icarus: Science and the Transformation of Contemporary Democracy* (Cambridge, Mass.: Harvard University Press, 1990).

13. President's Commission for the Study of Ethical Problems in Medicine and Biomedical and Behavioral Research, *Splicing Life: A Report on the Social and Ethical Issues of Genetic Engineering with Human Beings* (Washington, D.C.: U.S. Government Printing Office, 1983).

14. This research is elaborated further in John H. Evans, *Playing God? Human Genetic Engineering and the Rationalization of Public Bioethical Debate, 1959–1995* (Chicago: University of Chicago Press, 2001).

15. Letter from Leon Kass to Alexander Capron, Executive Director, President's Commission for the Study of Ethical Problems in Medicine and Biomedical and Behavioral Research, 7 April 1981 (emphasis in original). Archived in the Archives of the President's Commission, National Bioethics Reference Center, Georgetown University, Washington, D.C.

16. This is the problem of incommensurable values. For a more extensive discussion from a philosophical perspective, see Elizabeth Anderson, *Value in*

Ethics and Economics (Cambridge, Mass.: Harvard University Press, 1993); Margaret Radin, *Contested Commodities* (Cambridge, Mass.: Harvard University Press, 1996). For a sociological perspective, see Wendy Nelson Espeland and Mitchell L. Stevens, "Commensuration as a Social Process," *Annual Review of Sociology* 24 (1998): 313–31.

17. Ezrahi, *The Descent of Icarus*, p. 91.

18. Wendy Espeland, *The Struggle for Water: Politics, Rationality and Identity in the American Southwest* (Chicago: University of Chicago Press, 1998), p. 25.

19. Erik Parens calls this the "argument from precedent" and notes its pervasive and questionable use in bioethics. Erik Parens, "Should We Hold the (Germ) Line?" *Journal of Law, Medicine and Ethics* 23 (1995): 173–76.

20. I will use the United Methodist Church as an example from this point forward simply because they are the religious group with the greatest amount of material available that explains their position.

21. In economics arguments, this is somewhat akin to the problem of arguing against negative externalities. The costs to individuals who lose their employment when a polluting factory is forcibly closed cannot be easily compared to the small costs each person in the region incurs due to the pollution.

22. Milton J. Coalter, John M. Mulder, and Louis B. Weeks, *Vital Signs: The Promise of Mainstream Protestantism* (Grand Rapids, Mich.: Williams B. Eerdmans Publishing, Co., 1996), p. 108.

23. Coalter, Mulder, and Weeks, *Vital Signs*, p. 108.

24. George Poste, "The Case for Genomic Patenting," *Nature* 378 (1995): 534–36, at 535.

25. George Poste, David Roberts, and Simon Gentry, "Patents, Ethics and Improving Healthcare," *Bulletin of Medical Ethics* (January 1997): 29–31, at 31.

26. Poste, Roberts, and Gentry, "Patents, Ethics, and Improving Healthcare," p. 31.

27. Poste, Roberts, and Gentry, "Patents, Ethics and Improving Healthcare," p. 31.

28. Stout, *Ethics After Babel*.

29. Unfortunately, these people are rare, and translation takes a lot of thinking through before presentation. This apparently did not happen in the gene patenting debate. See Mark J. Hanson, "Lessons from a Religious Objection to Genetic Patenting," in *Perspectives on Genetic Patenting: Religion, Science, and Industry in Dialogue*, ed. Audrey R. Chapman (Washington, D.C.: American Association for the Advancement of Science, 1999), pp. 221–34.

30. Jeffrey C. Alexander and Philip Smith, "The Discourse of American Civil Society: A New Proposal for Cultural Studies," *Theory and Society* 22 (1993): 151–207.

31. For a similar conclusion on translation, albeit from a somewhat different perspective than mine, see Ben C. Mitchell, "Is Moral Ambiguity All We Have to Offer?" *Christian Scholars Review* 23 (1994): 318–28.

32. Evans, "Playing God?"

33. There is of course a lot of discourse produced by bioethicists about abortion, but it is little compared to the discourse produced by social movements and repeated in the press.

34. Miguel Angel Centeno, "The New Leviathan: The Dynamics and Limits of Technocracy," *Theory and Society* 22 (1993): 307–35.

35. Daniel M. Fox, "View the Second," *Hastings Center Report* 23, no. 6 (1993): S12–13.

36. Gustafson, "Moral Discourse about Medicine," p. 127.

MARK J. HANSON

Religious Voices in Biotechnology: The Case of Gene Patenting

Religious traditions have long had more than passing interest in the developments of biotechnology—particularly as regards human life. Given the degree to which DNA is seen to be central to species and individual identity and the powers we are now obtaining over it, this should be no surprise. Further, religious traditions have largely endorsed the purported goals of biotechnology: human health and well-being.

But on 18 May 1995, nearly 200 religious leaders joined with leading biotechnology critic Jeremy Rifkin in a press conference named the "Joint Appeal against Human and Animal Patenting," a move that many within the biotechnology industry could only interpret as seeking to inhibit biotechnological advance. What moral and religious concerns motivated this challenge to patenting? How could the biotechnology industry understand and respectfully attend to these concerns? What values were at play in the debates that followed the joint appeal? What lessons for future dialogue can be learned from attempts at conversation between the opposing positions?

This chapter is a report from a Hastings Center research project that accepted the task of addressing these questions. Specifically, the project focused on the patenting of human genetic material, a subset of the issues raised by the joint appeal.

While the U.S. Patent and Trademark Office might seem a strange place for religious leaders to make a stand, the issue of patenting brings together a wide variety of concerns regarding biotechnology, some of which reflect on patenting itself and some of which engage biotechnology more generally. I believe it would be a mistake to conclude, as many in the industry did (perhaps because of the association with Rifkin), that religious opposition to patenting was largely motivated by fear of future abuse or moral transgression by biotechnology companies. While these fears indeed exist—along with other concerns about eugenics and corporate control of biotechnological resources—religious opposition to patenting itself also reflects concerns that are ethically noteworthy and often echoed in nonreligious critiques.[1] Thus a major purpose of this chapter is to demonstrate that patenting is indeed an ethical issue, not simply an economic one as asserted by the Biotechnology Industry Organization (BIO),[2] or a legal one as stated by the director of the Human Genome Project at the National Institutes of Health, Francis Collins.[3]

In the end, I do not believe that the religious objections to gene patenting are sufficient on balance to warrant a full ban on all such patents, although certain patents—such as on engineered human embryos—would be objectionable. Moreover, there is room for further exploration of ethically preferable alternatives to current patent law.

The primary task of this chapter, however, is to take the preliminary step of putting forward the values motivating this debate—especially what seems to be at stake for religious critics—in the ethically richest manner possible. Dialogues among interested parties since the joint appeal have demonstrated a certain "thinness" with regard to the range of values and worldviews at play, resulting in a general frustration of participants talking past each other. I will also provide analysis of the discussions following the May 1995 appeal and extrapolate some lessons for future dialogue at the intersection of religion and biotechnology. I hope that increasing the understanding of the complexity of the issues raised, in itself, will not only contribute to a more constructive dialogue at the intersection of religion and biotechnology, but ultimately lead toward more responsible ethics and policy in biotechnology itself.

Before proceeding to an analysis of these concerns, it is important to consider the context in which they are raised and how they are currently being expressed.

A Brief Background

By the time of the joint appeal in 1995 it had been fifteen years since the Supreme Court ruled in *Diamond v. Chakrabarty* that a genetically engineered micro-organism was patentable subject matter. For many commentators, the Court's five-to-four decision in *Chakrabarty* represented a fundamental change in interpretation of patent law. While phenomena of nature are not patentable, for the first time the Court interpreted this as not encompassing phenomena of nature in which there had been some human intervention that satisfied the criteria for patentability, namely, that the subject matter is novel, useful, and nonobvious. The decision prompted some discussion in bioethics circles but was little noticed among religious groups. And according to a 1989 report by the Office of Technology Assessment, early critics of gene patenting focused their objections on the potential uses and risks of biotechnology generally, rather than patenting per se.[4]

Although theologians had been among the leaders in public discussions of genetics in the 1970s, most religious organizations did not respond to genetic science until the 1980s, when reports were issued by the World Council of Churches, the National Council of the Churches of Christ in the U.S.A., the Roman Catholic Church, a few U.S. Protestant denominations, and a smattering of Christian churches abroad.[5] Although there are differences among the documents, they generally support—albeit with due caution—the potential for genetic technologies to improve human health and well-being. Just what limits are to be imposed, and on which theological and ethical bases, were, at best, ambiguously delineated.

But certain lines in the sand had been drawn prior to the 1995 joint appeal, which was not the first time religious leaders had joined together to make their views known on genetic technologies. In 1983 fifty religious leaders also collaborated with Rifkin to sign a resolution to oppose "efforts to engineer specific genetic traits in the germline of the human species."[6] This was followed four years later with a similar effort opposing the patenting of genetically engineered animals, such as the so-called Harvard oncomouse.

In 1992 the United Methodist Church task force on genetics issued a wide-ranging report to the Church's general conference, identifying theological concerns with the patenting of genes and concluding that "genes and genetically modified organisms (human, plant, animal) be held as common resources and not be exclusively controlled or patented."[7] After the U.S. Patent and Trademark Office issued patents on two transgenic mice, the Methodist Church made contact with Rifkin and other religious groups about the issue. Rifkin then became instrumental in building the coalition that issued the 1995 joint appeal.

Although much of the media coverage of the joint appeal press conference characterized the event in terms of science versus religion,[8] it is important to recognize the ways in which that was not the case. First, religious leaders were careful to reiterate—at the press conference and in other documents—that they support the general goals of biotechnology and are not opposed to the industry's drive for profits. Second, subsequent discussion among religious leaders and theologians has revealed a great deal of disagreement among religionists about patenting of biological materials. And third, the stance against gene patenting by professional groups of scientists such as the Council for Responsible Genetics demonstrates a lack of unanimity among the scientific and industrial communities as well.

The debate today has taken on a different character from earlier discussions. Although general concerns about biotechnology may still motivate critics of gene patenting, the recent debates make more explicit reference to the ethical, religious, and cultural commitments of the participants, as Mark Sagoff has noted.[9] The major difficulty in making the move from such rich references to constructive conversation, however, has been the limited way in which these commitments have been developed and explicated. A quick map of the terrain will set up my analysis of these issues.

The gene patenting debate engages values from three spheres: religion, biotechnology, and the law. It is important to note that while one may distinguish the values and world views at work within each sphere for the purpose of analysis, these spheres are composed of people who hold various blends of perspectives. To begin to see how diverse perspectives played out in the debate, however, we must begin with the assumptions that motivate this controversy (and likely future controversies), namely, how DNA—the material responsible for transmitting hereditary characteristics—is understood. Is it sacred? Is it merely a chemical compound? Is it wholly or only partially intertwined with human (or other species) identity?

In the recent debates on gene patenting, answers to these questions have led to additional points of controversy. If DNA does have a special nature given its role in determining identity, does patenting DNA sequences violate that nature in such a way that patenting should be limited or even prohibited? Religious critics have raised the argument that patenting entails a way of valuing genetic material that is inappropriate: DNA is not the kind of thing that should be owned; it should not be controlled by biotechnology companies in the ways patenting enables; and it should not be commodified. For religious critics, these arguments are ultimately all of a piece. Yet religionists still have much work to do to make sense of the implication of biotechnology in the context of their traditions. My analysis will try to fill in these arguments more fully and establish connections with a more secular articulation of the issues.

For the biotechnology industry, the dominant values at stake are the help their products can bring people in terms of health and well-being, and the economic survival of their industry. The perceived necessity of gene patents to serve these goods entails a different perspective on how DNA ought to be valued: it is a chemical compound, even if it is unlike other chemicals in relation to human identity. This narrow view of DNA and the range of values at stake in this controversy stands in obvious tension with the claims of the religious critics.

These perspectives clash over a matter of law, the patentability of genetic material that has been the object of some human inventive step. Although in the legal sphere patents are merely mechanisms to establish a certain bundle of rights that exclude others from making, using, or selling the patented subject matter, there are values implicit in the criteria for establishing patentability, such as what can be patented and why. These values also come into play in the gene patenting debate.

The literature and dialogue on the gene patenting issue to date have displayed how easily those of diverse perspectives misunderstand each other. The substance of the issues involved and modes of communication utilized in this controversy make it an instructive case study for many future debates regarding developments in biotechnology.

The Meaning of DNA

At the heart of the gene patenting controversy is ultimately the question: What are genes (and their components) that makes them unique from other matter such that patenting them would cause public controversy?

In defending patenting, representatives of the biotechnology industry have generally insisted on describing genes and DNA as mere chemical compounds, a definition that is reinforced by the language of legal decisions regarding gene patenting.[10] By minimizing the significance of DNA, patent defenders hope to minimize the possible moral offense that others could take at the practice. To state this is to note that the rhetoric used to describe DNA often varies with the context in which it is discussed.

Yet geneticists have also described DNA in terms that characterize it in much more ethically significant terms than "mere chemical." In their book *The DNA Mystique: The Gene as Cultural Icon*, sociologist Dorothy Nelkin and historian Susan Lindee describe how scientists have described DNA as the "Bible," the "Book of Man," and the "Holy Grail."[11] Such language grants power and prestige to the scientists who work with such material and may be rhetorically useful for attracting capital investment in their work.

The use of "religious" language by scientists also suits the media and popular culture, which are tantalized by the suggestion of finding the biological key to the mysteries of human nature and even immortality. According to Nelkin and Lindee, "the cultural depiction of DNA shares many characteristics with the immortal soul of Christianity. . . . DNA is relatively independent of the body, gives the body life and power, and is the point at which true identity (and self) can be determined."[12] In this way, DNA has assumed a sacred quality; tampering or even patenting it violates its sacredness and truly puts human scientists in the position of playing God.

Nelkin and Lindee acknowledge the genetic essentialism captured in this kind of talk—equating genes with human essence. And while such essentialism may be in fact contrary to the professed doctrines of many religious traditions, it nevertheless is easily derived from them. It can thus take a strong hold on the popular imagination and forms of discourse:

> The gene has become a way to talk about the boundaries of personhood, the nature of immortality, and the sacred meaning of life in ways that parallel theological narratives. Just as the Christian soul has provided an archetypal concept through which to understand the persona and the continuity of the self, so DNA appears in popular culture as a soul-like entity, a holy and immortal relic, a forbidden territory.[13]

Far from being merely metaphorical, Nelkin and Lindee add that DNA has in fact taken on the "social and cultural functions of the soul. It is the essential entity—the location of the true self—in the narratives of biological determinism."[14] By importing religious language into the context of genetic technology, biotechnology has invited this kind of genetic essentialism; there can be no surprise that religious groups would take interest in the subject.

While many religious leaders and theologians also deny a genetic essentialism, the patenting issue demonstrates that for religious critics of gene patenting, genes possess characteristics integral to human identity and personhood. More than that, some religious leaders have accepted the view of DNA as sacred. Among certain Christian critics, DNA provides the biological blueprint for human beings as the image of God. It thus possesses a special kind of intrinsic value that makes patenting of it inappropriate.

Because these arguments are central to the religious objections, I will develop these claims in more detail below. What the range of interpretations of genes and DNA demonstrates, however, is that definitions reflect broader traditions of interpreting reality. While those definitions can be engaged by persons outside those traditions, simply to assert alternative definitions does not contribute to constructive dialogue.

The Values of the United States Patent System

In response to the joint appeal, there was a concerted effort by the Patent and Trademark Office (PTO) as well as the biotechnology industry to explain the nature and scope of patents. This effort was motivated by the assumption that many critics misunderstand patents. While this may be true in some cases, it is also important to note that defenders of gene patents employ a minimalist understanding that fails to attend to certain features of patents, the symbolic implications of patenting, and the expressive function of patent law in a society. In short, while some critics of patents may not understand patents and patent rights adequately, defenders of patents for biological materials may be faulted for a fundamentally similar shortcoming.

Much of the puzzlement by industry and representatives of the PTO over the religious leaders' objections to certain patents stems from understanding of patents as "mere mechanisms" to encourage investment and promote research. Yet patents themselves—in their purposes, their ethical justifications, and how they are interpreted and applied—are not "mere mechanisms." There is a more expansive way to understand the values implied by the patent system and the way patents are currently interpreted by the PTO.

The minimal definition of patents is roughly as follows: A patent is a form of intellectual property rights granted in reference to an invention only if it meets three criteria: it must be useful, novel, and nonobvious. I consider the criterion of usefulness (or utility) below but note here that it excludes that which is merely an object of curiosity or research. By "novel" is meant that "the subject matter as claimed did not previously exist either as described in a publication or in physical form."[15] Patents are not allowed, therefore, on phenomena or laws of nature without some inventive step. "Nonobviousness" relates to whether the "subject matter as a whole would have been obvious at the time the invention was made to a person having ordinary skill in the art to which said subject matter pertains" (35 U.S. Code §103).

As a bundle of exclusionary intellectual property rights, a patent prohibits others from making, using, or selling the patented subject matter for a limited period of time (twenty years from the date of issue). Further, as a form of intellectual property, a patent must define the subject matter. The nature of patent rights as "merely" exclusionary makes them less comprehensive than full ownership rights. As a result, most defenders of patents for genes and other biological materials are adamant to claim that patents do not confer ownership upon the patented subject matter. The right to exclude does not include the right to utilize the invention (as would ownership rights); such practice would be subject to other relevant regulations. The issue of "ownership," however, is contentious and more than simply a point of legal subtlety.

For defenders of patents on genes, patents are legal instruments with an economic function. They confer a bundle of rights that functions as a mechanism for promoting investment in biotechnology and its goals. Any further interpretation, on their view, is either a misunderstanding or an "overreading" of the meaning of patents. But this understanding of patents is inadequate to account for both the other values that inhere in patents and the controversy about them.

In his book *Toward a More Natural Science*, Leon Kass notes the significance of the value of scientific and technological progress for the American Founders.[16] The U.S. patent system is grounded in the Constitution itself: "The Congress shall have Power . . . To promote the Progress of Science and useful Arts, by securing for limited Times to Authors and Inventors the exclusive Right to their respective Writings and Discoveries" (Article I, Sec. 8).

But as Kass argues, progress for its own sake was not the final goal. Congress was to provide for the useful arts, and the utility of those arts was defined by Madison in the *Federalist* (No. 43) in terms of the public good. Patents and copyrights were to be instituted to provide incentives to inventors to develop knowledge and discoveries in service of the goals of the American democracy.

Kass's analysis also discloses the extent to which patent law is a matter of morality, in terms of both justice and character:

> [E]veryone sees the at least prima facie claim that justice requires protecting the labors of the imaginative and industrious against theft by the sly and lazy. If theft of property is wrong, the right of patent is right, at least to some extent. The foundation of the patent law is not only utilitarian, but also ethical. Indeed, it is ethical also in its consequences for character.

The law not only protects individual rights and prevents injustice; it also rewards and encourages the energetic cultivation of the mind and the intellectual virtues of inventiveness, order, and precision, and promotes, in publicly beneficial ways, the moral virtues of ambition and industry.[17]

The purely utilitarian features of the patent system receive the most attention from defenders of patents on biological materials: patents encourage research and development, which in turn promotes innovative production of goods and services that may serve social goods in addition to scientific and economic progress. For the biotechnology industry, these features of patents are employed in argument on behalf of the ends of the industry itself and are not seen by them as ethical in their own right. The core argument (detailed below) is that only patent protection can sufficiently encourage financial investment in the technologies needed to develop products that save lives and promote health. Patents are merely the mechanism to promote these ends.

The justifiability of the research and patent on resulting products is taken for granted. Yet it is precisely on this point that critics of patents on biotechnologies re-enter the picture. While critics may concede that a patent on a particular product may, in fact, promote a valuable public good—such as health—their criticisms of patents in certain cases constitute a challenge that patents, as well as certain technologies, may not always promote the public good. Cases in biotechnology in particular may highlight difficult tensions in patent law.[18] Unlike the European Patent Convention, which prohibits patents for inventions "the publication or exploitation of which would be contrary to public order or morality" (Article 53[a]), the U.S. patent system contains no explicit provision for evaluation of what the Constitution called "progress" in terms of the public good. Only the criterion of usefulness allows, at least potentially, for some degree of value judgment.

Through much of the history of decisions regarding patent applications, the criterion of usefulness seems to be ill defined. In fact, it seems largely assumed by the PTO that no one would bother with the trouble and expense of the patent application unless the usefulness criterion were satisfied. More recent commentary, however, has noted the extent to which this criterion is interpreted in terms of economic values. According to attorney E. Richard Gold, "The United States Supreme Court has held that a discovery that is 'useful' only in the sense that it is of scientific interest—such as a new compound health researchers wish to investigate for tumor-inhibiting effects—does not qualify as being useful under the statute."[19] On Gold's interpretation

the Court disavows competency to take account of other values—
such as effects on health, environment, or human dignity—which only
Congress should address.[20] Lacking a more expansive definition of usefulness and/or an added criterion for morality, the patent office will be
of limited service in setting boundaries on the inventions of science
and technology with regard to the public good, despite the ethical load
that patents themselves carry.

A further point where values are implicit in the patent system arises
on the question of what constitutes patentable subject matter. Assuming
other criteria are met, the U.S. patent code authorizes patent protection
for the invention or discovery of "any new and useful process, machine,
manufacture, or composition of matter, or any new and useful improve-
ment thereof" (35 U.S. Code §101). Two points are important: first,
the Court's decision in *Chakrabarty* demonstrates that the status of an
organism as living is irrelevant to patentability. As long as some intervention is accomplished that satisfies the patent code's criteria, a patent is
justified. This is important to consider given religious arguments aimed
at safeguarding the "sacredness of life." Second, PTO decisions since
Chakrabarty have considered DNA sequences as mere chemical compounds, patentable as compositions of matter if they are isolated and
purified.[21] This raises the issue of how one understands DNA, a question
at the core of the patent controversy. As I will consider, the question
of what constitutes patentable subject matter is hardly a neutral or
benign component of the law.

The significant presence of ethically relevant values in the patent
system also parallels one further consideration regarding the role of the
law in the debates about the patenting of genetic materials, and that is
its general expressive function in society. Much has been written about
the various functions of law within societies. One feature of this discussion that the patenting controversy brings to prominence, however, is
the law's expressive power in relation to a society's basic values and
character. Particularly in a culture as strongly oriented toward the law
as the United States, where many significant moral issues are settled
within the courts, the power of the law to shape the moral character
of a society is enormous. Law can be understood as part of the constitutive rhetoric of our communities; it helps shape our understanding of
ourselves and our relations to each other.[22] That we would consider
genetic material or biological organisms subject to patent law—interpreted as it is largely in terms of economic value applied to certain conceptions of "manufacture" and "compositions of matter"—does not merely

witness to our values of promoting investment in biotechnology; it also testifies to the way in which the society defines and values the patented subject matter. Put more strongly, "legal instantiation changes the thing itself."[23] In other words, once DNA is codified in particular terms as a human invention, the public understanding of it is changed. Thus merely repeating the letter of the law on patents will not suffice to explain how a particular patent may be understood by certain social groups whose dominant interests and values are ultimately not those of invention and economic self-interest. I believe this to be largely accountable for the response of religious communities to the patenting of biological materials.

The Values of the Biotechnology Industry

The biotechnology industry's response to the joint appeal—particularly through its major umbrella groups, the Biotechnology Industry Organization (BIO) and the Pharmaceutical Research and Manufacturers of America (PhRMA)—was swift and consistent. Their defense of patents reveals clusters of values that fall into three general types of argument: self-interest, utility, and desert, with the utilitarian argument providing the major burden of justification and the other arguments at times also invoked in service of utility.

Self-Interest

While the argument from self-interest alone would not be seen by many as a moral argument (insofar as it lacks an other-regarding component), clearly the biotechnology industry defends patents because it believes them to be necessary for its economic self-interest. Quite distinct from broader ethical claims, patents are seen as a necessary legal mechanism for encouraging the investment of capital into companies and protecting the results of research from competition until such investments can achieve and maximize a financial return. "Patents are a fundamental element of our free enterprise system," asserts BIO.[24] More to the point, SmithKline Beecham Pharmaceutical's Chairman of Research and Development, George Poste, concluded, "For industrial participants, the motivation [for responding to debate about patents], unsurprisingly, is the quest for commercial leadership in genetic medicine."[25]

While arguments from economic self-interest play a relatively minor role in the public defense of patents, the presence of a profit motive invites a measure of skepticism from critics insofar as it provides an inevitable but unavoidable obstacle to trust. Yet the profit motive and moral justification may, obviously, also coincide in support of the same ends, as the industry often claims.

Utility

I have already noted the general utilitarian justification for patents. For the biotechnology industry, the same general ends apply: incentive for research and development; enhanced competitiveness, which in turn catalyzes "depth and breadth in research innovation";[26] openness regarding research developments; and scientific as well as economic progress. These ends are ultimately subsumed to the overarching moral ends and ostensible justifications for biotechnology itself, namely, prevention of suffering and promotion of health and well-being.

BIO and PhRMA ground their strongest appeal on the issue of suffering. In fact, BIO took the curious position that patenting only becomes an ethical issue when laws against patenting are enacted. When patenting is obstructed, "research will not be funded or advanced and patients will continue to suffer."[27] Such arguments simultaneously locate those who support patents outside of morality, in the supposedly ethically neutral realms of law and economics, and characterize those who would deny patents as immoral. Three representatives of SmithKline Beecham echoed these sentiments when they argued that denying patents "would betray the moral obligation to relieve suffering and would be deeply unethical."[28] PhRMA's press release following the joint appeal makes the boldest case for biotechnology and the need for patents to ensure its success:

> Biotechnology holds out the promise of a new Golden Age of Medicine. This nascent science allows researchers to intervene in the disease process. Many medicines available today would not be possible without patents on genetically altered material. . . . Prohibiting current patent practices for genetic engineering, as urged, would deprive millions of people of even the hope of a cure through biotechnology.[29]

Finally, an argument has also been made that patents in biotechnology ultimately save money and can help keep down health care costs.[30] For instance, a drug for peptic ulcers now replaces expensive surgery.

Desert

A final value reflected in the industry argument on behalf of patents reflects the justice argument for patents generally, namely, that patents ensure just reward for contributions and efforts. In other words, it would be unfair if there were no mechanism for ensuring that investment of capital and labor had opportunity for reward, or if those who did not contribute to the invention could capitalize on the products of investments without contributing to them or compensating the inventors. While reward is a value in its own right, it also is instrumental in the larger utilitarian argument for patents. The promise of these rewards provides the incentives for further advance.

Yet the biotechnology industry's defense of patents is not unproblematic. It is beyond the scope of this essay to review and analyze all possible arguments related to gene patenting. A couple of points are worth making, however, as they relate to the religious concerns.

First, no objections have been raised by religious leaders regarding the justification of patents in general or the ends served by biotechnology patents in particular. Religious critics grant even the self-interest of the industry as instrumental to promoting the industry's goals of human economic and biological well-being and therefore justified. Rather, concerns are related to how patents on genes and other biological entities may impinge on other values not recognized by the industry, and whether there aren't ethically preferable alternatives that would still accomplish the industry's goals.

Second, in this respect it is worth noting the existence of a secular literature that particularly challenges the utilitarian arguments for patents in light of possible alternatives. Michele Svatos, for instance, notes a number of drawbacks to patents as a tool for promoting incentives.[31] These include "inefficient allocation of resources, encouragement of 'work-arounds' or copycat inventions, changes in the allocation of research funds, increased secrecy, substantial legal and administrative costs, an arbitrary focus on the sorts of research which are patentable, and differential effects depending on the stage of industry development" (p. 117). In short, patents create their own difficulties for research and business, making the current system far from perfect. Even ardent patent defenders will admit to problems entailed by the current patent system, including the millions of dollars spent each year on patent litigation. Alternatives to the current system have also been suggested but remain largely undeveloped.

In addition, the cost-effectiveness of biotechnology remains uncertain. In a new era of technology assessment and managed care, biotechnology is coming increasingly under scrutiny for its long-term cost-effectiveness. The history of rising health care costs has shown the dubiousness of the common argument that new technologies will save money in the long run. Moreover, biotechnology products are particularly expensive to develop and have high acquisition costs. Given these expenses and the high degree of uncertainty surrounding many biotechnology investments, the special difficulties biotechnology brings to the new wave of technology assessment require further investigation before the industry's argument for cost-effectiveness can be granted.[32]

Ultimately, however, the problems with the industry's defense relate less to the arguments made and more to the lack of recognition of the values raised up by critics. It is to these values that I now turn.

The Values of Religious Traditions in Their Objections to Gene Patenting

That the May 1995 joint appeal captured such wide support across the spectrum of American religious traditions is remarkable. Not only did the signatories agree on the statement as a conclusion to their consideration of the issue; subsequent dialogue has shown a general unity among leading critics on the types of arguments utilized in support of the statement. My analysis will address the common themes.

As a caveat, however, it is important to note that the "religious leaders" who signed the appeal were not generally representing official positions of their denominations. In addition, there is significant disagreement among members of some traditions that are represented. Thus it would be a mistake to conclude that the joint appeal represents rare unanimity. In fact, some of the most productive dialogue and liveliest debate in the wake of the appeal have been among theologians and church leaders on the theological issues raised by patenting.

I have suggested that the religious response to patenting of biological materials is not motivated entirely, or even largely, by fear of biotechnology or abuse of it in the future. Certainly there are echoes of such concerns within various statements by religious leaders. For example, at his National Press Club statement, Dr. Richard Land, president of the Southern Baptist Convention's Christian Life Commission, characterized the altering or creation of life forms "as a revolt against God's sovereignty and the attempt by humankind to usurp God and be God."[33] Such a concern, generally speaking, is not unique to adherents of religious traditions; indeed, it is expressed in different terms within secular advocacy groups and the biotechnology industry as well (for example, the Council for Responsible Genetics).

The dominant theme of various statements and written work opposing patenting of genetic and other biological materials is how patenting places these materials, broadly speaking, in the realm of the marketplace. In the eyes of the critics, this move necessarily implies an understanding and valuation that is inappropriate and thus should be prohibited.

My analysis indicates that while the theological bases for many of the concerns raised by religious leaders remain mostly inadequately articulated, several of their arguments reflect ethically legitimate concerns that deserve further attention and exploration. Although the theological objections to patenting seem too thin to justify a ban on patents for genetic material—as many theologians themselves conclude—further mutual accommodation in both the terms of the debate and modification of patent policy may be possible. Such accommodations should continue to be explored.

Ownership

A major objection to biological patenting common to leaders of the joint appeal coalition involves the issue of ownership. The basic argument is succinctly stated by Richard Land and C. Ben Mitchell of the Southern Baptist Convention's Christian Life Commission:

> Human beings are pre-owned. We belong to the sovereign Creator. We are, therefore, not to be killed without adequate justification (e.g., in self-defense) nor are we, or our body parts, to be bought and sold in the marketplace. Yet, the patenting of human genetic material attempts to wrest ownership from God and commodifies human biological materials and, potentially, human beings themselves. Admittedly, a single human gene or a cell line is not a human being; but a human gene or cell line is undeniably human and warrants different treatment than all non-human genes or cell lines. The image of God pervades human life in all of its parts. Furthermore, the right to own one part of a human being is ceteris paribus the right to own all the parts of a human being. This right must not be transferred from the Creator to the creature.[34]

This kind of argument raises several issues that have been challenged on both legal and theological grounds.

In response to these arguments, representatives from the PTO and the biotechnology industry have been quick to argue that patents do not entail ownership. Full ownership rights, it is argued, confer rights of use or disposal that are limited only by other pertinent regulations. Patent rights, on the other hand, are more restrictive: they are prohibitive or exclusionary regarding commercial exploitation of an invention.

Furthermore, the patent right does not extend to any biological material that exists inside a living being. Thus it would be incorrect to claim that a patent holder "owns," for instance, a part of someone's or anyone's body.

But while the technical understanding of the term ownership may be defined to accomplish certain legal functions or to avoid certain legal and ethical difficulties, there are two points regarding the critics' (continued) use of the term that are ethically significant. First, it is not fully established that the use of the term ownership with regard to patents is in error. Ownership is most commonly defined as a "bundle of rights" that can admit of degrees. As philosopher Judith Andre notes, "I can own a sewing machine more completely than I can own historic buildings."[35] In other words, there are greater and lesser bundles of rights that still constitute ownership, and precise boundaries of the concept are difficult to determine.[36] In addition, frequent use of the term with regard to patents by persons from a variety of disciplines demonstrates that its application to patent rights is not inconsistent with many persons' general understanding of what can be encompassed by ownership.[37]

Second, even if the technical, legal definition of ownership can be strictly defined in favor of the patent defenders' interpretation, it is noteworthy that the term continues to be employed by critics, even though the "correct" definition of patents has been explained. More importantly, it seems to be the case that critics are not using the term strictly according to its legal function but rather as a symbolic placeholder for a certain set of moral and religious arguments to which common notions of ownership are distinctly related.

What are these arguments? They have not been articulated systematically or at any great length, but the invocation of "ownership" seems to combine three sets of interrelated claims. The first regards the unique status of DNA or the biological materials in question and how their status makes them an inappropriate subject matter for any bundle of "proprietary" rights, including rights to restrict access to the patented materials. These considerations, then, also enable a set of claims regarding how patenting challenges important ultimate questions of sovereignty in concerns about the nature of power and control over DNA and genetic information. And finally, ownership language is used to highlight the central objection of patenting as commodification, insofar as ownership and commodification are closely related in common discourse.

In the case of human genes, Land and Mitchell begin their argument against "ownership" as follows: "Opposition to patenting Homo sapiens and their genetic parts is grounded in the unique nature of human beings. Human beings, alone among living organisms, bear the *imago Dei* [image of God]."[38] Thus even though a human being may share up to 95 percent of his or her genetic material with a nonhuman species, the "image of God pervades human life in all of its parts."[39] Presumably, any gene that belongs to the human genome, even if identical to genes of other species, has a status that is unique, intrinsically valuable, and, according to some, sacred. Furthermore, all life, as created by God and thus a gift of God, has intrinsic value. Although genes are not alive, they are recognized as the "building blocks of life" and thus so intimately related to life that treatment of genes is in moral respects identical with treatment of life itself.[40]

The use of ownership language by critics, then, attempts to communicate the message that patenting is inappropriate because genetic material is not the kind of thing that could and/or should be subject to any kind of proprietary rights. Drawing on a distinction by philosopher Paul Thompson, Audrey Chapman, director of the Dialogue Program between Science and Religion at the American Association for the Advancement of Science, rightly notes that critics are employing an "ontological conception of property," which "bases property status on traits or characteristics alleged to inhere in specific objects," thereby excluding certain categories of objects from property claims.[41] This is to be distinguished from the "instrumental" conception of property employed by patent defenders, which characterizes property as a "legal fiction, an artifact or a legal code, which is validated to the extent that it is useful in promoting some more fundamental social, political, or economic end."[42]

Given this ontological usage employed by critics, Judith Andre's discussion of ownership is again illuminating. Among those things which by their nature cannot be owned are divine grace or gifts from God: "An omnipotent God is beyond the reach of the state. It is meaningless to talk of protecting with force one's status before God. The reason one cannot sell divine grace is that one does not own it to begin with."[43]

If one understands DNA to be a building block of life, a gift from God—bearing, in a sense, the grace of God—it would not be the sort of thing that proprietary rights of any sort—even those short of full ownership—could or should apply to.

In addition, assertions by critics of patenting that genes are the common heritage of humanity place genetic material in a further category of things that cannot be owned, namely, as Andre notes, when "the use of some things cannot be confined to any individual or group."[44] So even if patenting does not confer ownership, Andre's analysis helps illustrate the sense people may have that certain things, by their nature, may be inappropriate subjects of any sort of proprietary discourse, including patenting. Use of the term ownership by critics serves to make this point more sharply in public rhetoric.

The second set of claims on which the ownership objection depends relates to the issue of sovereignty. Because of the special status of living things generally, and human beings especially, as created recipients of the gift of life, they are necessarily in relationship with the Creator. According to the critics, the creator's sovereignty over the creation is such that human beings may be thought of as "owned" by God, such that certain other forms of "ownership" are inappropriate.

What would it mean to be owned by God? The view that God's ownership entails a right to use, dispose, or alter any thing, and also to prohibit such activity by others, would be consistent with a narrow conception of ownership as well as certain (but not all) doctrines of God. But clearly, to be owned by God could not be strictly analogous to the relationship that human beings have with things that they own. While one might believe that all things "belong" to God, most religious traditions understand God to have given life as a gift to living creatures, and the rest of creation as gifts to be shared among creatures. Jewish and Christian traditions also believe that human beings have been given dominion over the rest of creation, within which they have established various systems of ownership.

So how might God's ownership be more accurately understood? Protestant theologian Ronald Cole-Turner argues that God's ownership of all things is best understood as God's reserving the right to define their purpose, value, and relationship to other creatures.

> God owns the land, not to exclude creatures from it, but to give it for their right use and to set the limits of proper use and care. . . . Human beings may own individual animals and plants, and their components may be bought, sold, and used for food. That is, we may own these things as long as God's prior claim of ownership is acknowledged, as long as we own them in a way that is consistent with God's definition of their purpose. It is wrong to own any of these things in a way that denies God's prior ownership.[45]

Cole-Turner does not believe that patenting itself could violate this sense of God's ownership—although certain forms of genetic engineering, such as the Harvard oncomouse, would. I believe his conclusion to be correct. But I would argue that the invocation of ownership by critics stands primarily as an objection to the sense in which patenting implies a certain sovereignty over the patented subject matter that is theologically troublesome. How does it do this?

Judith Andre observes that "property is not a relation between a person and an object. It is a relation among people about that object."[46] Similarly, the ownership objection may offer critics of biological patents a way to assert that patents, as claims of corporate control, symbolize a denial of the sovereignty of God over life and those processes involved in its creation and modification. This may be how patents link up with what defenders believe is the deeper motivation for critics, namely, objection to biotechnologies themselves. Biotechnology does involve the hand of humanity in the creation and modification of life forms in a way that is more direct and efficient than more so-called natural processes, such as breeding. In short, it is one thing to be fruitful and multiply; it is another to be fruitful and modify. To claim this latter sort of power, the critics might assert, is to act as if one owned what is being manipulated.

Even though a patent does not legally entail usage rights, it claims for the patent holder a sovereignty over the information that enables the exercise of such power. In this sense, intellectual property rights may be more offensive to critics than full ownership rights. For example, the counterargument to the ownership objection has been that human beings own all sorts of living things, such as mules. Land and Mitchell invoke Leon Kass's argument in response that "It is one thing to own a mule; it is another to own mule."[47] The sense of species ownership invoked here is not the same as would apply if a person legally owned every mule in existence. Rather, what is objectionable is the intellectual property claim to sovereignty over the ideas that enable control over the creation of an entire and uniquely created species. The religious offense at the sovereignty implied by the "ownership" of these sorts of ideas—even for a limited time—is part of what the ownership objection is likely capturing. This argument, however, is obviously more powerful and relevant to the patenting of entire life forms than to genes or body parts.

The third set of claims that the ownership objection draws upon rests on the idea that patenting entails commodification. Because commodification has also been raised as a separate objection to patenting, I will deal with this as a separate heading.

Commodification

The commonest and most prominent objection to the patenting of biological materials was stated directly by Bishop Kenneth Carder of The United Methodist Church: "The issue . . . related to the patenting of genes is not science versus religion, nor is it opposition to biotechnology, nor denial of the necessity of economic return on capital investment. The issue is the commodification of life and the reduction of life to its commercial value and marketability."[48]

The issue of commodification is complex, and much has been written on it in relation to body parts of all kinds, particularly regarding markets for transplantation and sexual services. I cannot fully rehearse this literature here, but a couple of broad points illuminate the religious objection.

Does patenting entail commodification? Stanford University law professor Margaret Jane Radin distinguishes between narrow and broad senses of commodification.[49] The narrow sense applies only to the actual buying and selling of material goods and economic services. Regarding the narrow sense, patenting in itself would not seem to entail commodification in that patents do not involve commodity exchange. Furthermore, patents are certainly not a sufficient condition for ownership, which is the prerequisite to buying and selling. However, patents may be seen as related to the narrow sense of commodification in terms of what they enable, namely, the commercialization and possible monetary transaction involving genes and other biological material. That is, in today's biotechnology market, they seem to be a prerequisite for market transactions and the acquisition of profits that result from products that the patent enables. So while patents do not confer ownership, they are seen by critics of gene patenting as sufficiently and intimately linked to the context of market transactions that claims of ownership are invoked, even if these claims are ultimately misguided.

Yet Radin also identifies a broad understanding of commodification that encompasses market rhetoric even without exchange of material goods or services: "In market rhetoric, the discourse of commodification, one conceives of human attributes (properties of persons) as fungible owned objects (the property of persons). One conceives of human interactions as 'sales' with 'prices' even where no money literally changes hands."[50]

In other words, for the broad understanding of commodification to apply, the discourse must redescribe the object in market terms, whether or not the object is actually traded in the marketplace.

I suspect that what is at stake in the commodification objection—independent from any claims about ownership—relates to the market rhetoric described in this broad sense of commodification, namely, what Radin describes as universal commodification as a conceptual scheme or worldview. While, as she admits, universal commodification may be a caricature, it may nonetheless be useful for analysis:

From the perspective of universal commodification, all things desired or valued—from personal attributes to good government—are commodities. Anything that some people are willing to sell and that others are willing to buy can and should be in principle the subject of free market exchange.[51]

This world view, then, presents a "one dimensional world of value."[52] All features of reality come to be described in the common idiom of marketplace values, with nothing, in principle, excluded from possible exchange.

The patenting of DNA and genetically engineered life forms is seen by critics as another step in the advance of this world view. Patents are viewed as a form of market rhetoric applied to material—namely, DNA or engineered organisms—which possesses value that is nonreducible and religiously significant. Courts and the patent office become the targets of criticism insofar as they are the gatekeepers for the entrance of genetic material into the worldview of the market. What the commodification objection registers for critics of gene patents, then, is more a clash of world views than an objection that patents commodify genes in a narrow sense.

Moreover, as Radin points out, people are uncomfortable about market rhetoric because "it does tend to crystallize a social worry—the worry about inappropriate commodification" that is often linked to other kinds of social wrongs, such as injustice.[53] For example, our judgments about the morality of the selling of organs or babies often take account of the conditions of oppression that encourage such practices, as well as the harms that would accompany them. I will return to arguments about social injustice later.

Radin further argues that "the reason people are troubled by 'mere' market rhetoric, when applied in ways they think inappropriate, is that they think it will be 'contagious' and will lead to literal commodification."[54] We may recall Land and Mitchell's argument that "the principles, the reasoning, and the stance toward nature" invoked in the *Chakrabarty* decision may logically extend from bacteria to mules and beyond.[55] Further, Land's statement at the joint appeal includes a reference to the marketing of human life as a form of "genetic slavery."[56] Clearly, then, slippery slope arguments implied by Radin's description of universal commodification are part of the religious critics' concerns.

More broadly, the commodification objection is likely raised to signal objection to the way in which using market rhetoric in regard to genes seems to exclude noneconomic values and is therefore reductionistic. Although the justifications that patents promote health and well-being offered by the biotechnology industry may be endorsed by the critics, market reductionism nonetheless focuses more on the profits to be earned than the lives to be saved. Further, given how certain religious critics understand DNA, market rhetoric in itself becomes offensive as a primary mode of discourse in that it fails to value the genetic material appropriately. This perspective is powerfully reflected in Rabbi Saperstein's remarks at the joint appeal press briefing:

> We now see that [ultimate] value [of human life] degraded across our society—and we join together today in this broad coalition to raise our voices against the most fundamental degradation of all—the turning of all nature, perhaps even humanity itself, into an ownable market commodity. The patenting of life forms raises this issue directly and alarmingly.[57]

For Saperstein and many other religious critics, even if patents themselves do not commodify in a narrow sense, they "raise the issue" in the way that they contribute to a change in the terms of the discourse and thus a change in the way we value the patented subject matter.

The upshot is that the patenting of genes has contributed to what Radin calls "incomplete commodification," in both senses of that term.[58] Commodification is incomplete because not all segments of society accept genetic material as a commodity, and also because there may be a way to allow market and nonmarket understandings to coexist. Just as a person may consider a family heirloom to be priceless but also have its financial value assessed for insurance purposes, it is possible for competing and even conflicting world views and their rhetorics to coexist. If we can grant that there are multiple ways of valuing genetic material, that it is at minimum not "merely chemical," and that there may be some risk in complete commodification, we may all have a stake in maintaining incomplete commodification of that material. Prohibiting patenting is not necessary to accomplish this end. Nevertheless, I believe that the greatest value of the religious critics' objections to gene patenting lies in their "prophetic" role in maintaining an opposition to a complete crystallization of market rhetoric in relation to DNA. Even supporters of gene patents among theologians acknowledge this.[59]

Dignity

The relation of human dignity to the patenting of human genes, as such, has not been much addressed by religious critics of gene patenting. However, because the issue has been raised as an objection within various deliberations on the topic, and because it has been linked to commodification more specifically, I will make a couple points about it here.

As philosopher Baruch Brody's rich analysis of this topic indicates, this objection may take four forms: "ownership of human genes infringes on human dignity because it is equivalent to ownership of humans, because it commercializes body parts which should not be commodified, because it cheapens that which defines human identity, and because it would lead to inappropriate modifications in our genetic integrity."[60] Brody finds the first version of the argument to be unconvincing, primarily because as genes are patented they are external to the human body and also are not those of a particular human being. Ownership of something that "lacks a personal particularized connection either to me or to my body" is something altogether different from owning a person or a part of a person within that person's body. Thus, gene patenting does not violate human dignity in this way.

The second version of the dignity objection ties into concerns about commodification by providing an argument for why commodification of genes is objectionable, namely, because it violates human dignity. Yet as Brody points out, there are several ways in which the patenting of genes is disanalogous with the commodification of other body parts. Unlike the commercialization of organs for transplantation, genes are not removed from one person and placed in another for a price. There are thus no worries about exploitation of poor people or placing them at risk. Furthermore, gene patenting does not risk the same possible effects on the character of society by reducing possibilities for altruism. Dignity is not, therefore, reduced through commodification in these ways.

Brody, however, points to another way in which we might think of human dignity being compromised through gene patenting, namely, "by commodifying the very thing that defines our identity" (p. 11).[61] In support of this view, he points to the work of Mark Nelson, who related a principle that "it is wrong to sell something 'intimate' " to Radin's idea that "it is wrong to commercialize something with which individuality and personhood is intertwined."[62] This leads Brody to the third version of the dignity argument.

Questions of the meaning of individual identity and personhood have a complex history that cannot be rehearsed here. But Brody's cursory review of these questions leads him to what I believe is a defensible conclusion, namely, that the violation of human dignity through the commercialization of that with which individuality and personhood are intertwined would only apply to the patenting of a full set of genes—that is, the full, unique genome of a human individual. Therefore, the patenting of single, specific human gene would not impinge on dignity. Its commodification, on this reason, would not be objectionable.

The fourth version of the dignity objection, according to Brody, derives from the concern that human dignity could be disregarded through the commercialization of genetic modifications enabled by gene patenting. The more general concern is with preserving human genetic integrity, and among the likeliest bases for this, Brody believes, is the issue of eugenics. While the concern is, of course, reasonable, the objection would need to be strengthened through more precise parameters on what it would in fact prohibit. As it stands, attempts to apply the objection have been vague and have, in principle, ruled out too much.[63]

How would religious communities take account of these arguments? There is little in the statements of religious leaders to confirm or refute Brody's position explicitly. It is likely, however, that in contrast to Brody's analysis critics of gene patenting hold that what is "intimate" or intertwined with personal identity is not merely whole genomes but extends to individual genes, and thus that by commercializing such elements of identity gene patenting does significantly violate human dignity. This position derives from the particular view that "the image of God pervades human life in all of its parts."[64] It is the presence of this image that grants human beings their dignity, so the argument might go. Without being further refined and defended, both theologically and operationally as a basis for the rejection of gene patents, however, this argument remains problematic.

Reductionism

Another objection to gene patenting is that "patenting further identifies life mechanistically and blurs the distinction between the animate and the inanimate."[65] This objection is likely another way of articulating the sense that important ways of valuing genetic material and engineered life forms are being squeezed out of the public mind and discourse about genetics. So in addition to the reductionism of the market, there is a philosophical reductionism at work as well. In a commentary on the *Chakrabarty* decision, Leon Kass summarizes this view:

> [I]n [the Court's] eagerness to serve innovation, it has, perhaps unwittingly, become the teacher of philosophical materialism—the view that all forms are but accidents of underlying matter, that matter is what truly is—and therewith, the teacher also of the homogeneity of the given world, and, at least in principle, of the absence of any special dignity in all of living nature, our own included.[66]

This objection returns us to the issue of the meaning of DNA, and from my analysis it is clear that the issue is more complex than simply asserting in the face of this objection that DNA is not alive. How, then, does this materialism ground an objection to patenting? It may be here that concerns about the "expressive force" of law come importantly into play. That is, insofar as patenting necessarily involves treating "compositions of matter" in ways that do not attend to their status as living or as in any other way of transcendent value it also necessarily fosters the sort of philosophical materialism that critics find problematic.

Justice

To return, finally, to considerations of justice, the primary issue in this domain relates to the tension patents create between the (temporary) monopoly they grant to patent holders and equitable access to and distribution of the patented technology's benefits. The most fundamental objection, of course, would rest on a view of DNA as the common heritage of humanity—owned either by God, by none, or by all. In any case, to claim monopolistic control over even a bit of DNA is to commit an injustice by claiming for oneself—that is, the patent holder— something that rightfully "belongs" to others or to no one. Such concerns have been raised more often by secular organizations in relation to the patenting of biological material from indigenous peoples or from individuals possessing unique genetic "resources" for the development of medical treatments.[67]

A more frequent justice objection stems from how the monopoly created by patents centralizes corporate power and control over the products resulting from the patents, particularly how those products are priced and distributed. Even if patents on genetic material are accepted in principle, it has been argued that some compensation is due those who served as sources of the genetic material.

Overall, justice concerns have been secondary among the objections raised by religious leaders, insofar as justice is more of an issue that follows as a consequence of patenting—how patents are used—rather than an intrinsic argument about the morality of the patent itself. Religious institutions have long been sensitive to circumstances of injustice, however, and have played a critical social role—through prophetic discourse as well as in ethics and policy dialogue—in identifying injustice and promoting social justice.

Summary Analysis of the Religious Objections

In the preceding section I have tried to uncover and make the best ethical sense of the values embedded in the religious objections to gene patenting. This task illustrates the difficulty of evaluating objections as they have been articulated in religious statements and published material, given that this debate is essentially what Audrey Chapman has called a "theology in process."[68] It is, therefore, more difficult to analyze than to contribute to further understanding. I can make a few broad critical observations regarding the religious objections at this point.

First, the conceptions of DNA that underlie the religious critics' objections based on ownership—especially the claims that genes are sacred and that even human DNA fragments bear the image of God— are theologically underdeveloped and ultimately problematic. Because of the ease with which the term sacred can be used to set religious and ethical boundaries, its meaning should be carefully defined and its use well defended. This was not done in this case. Further, applying the term sacred to DNA fragments may end up prohibiting too much, a justified concern for the biotechnology industry and a source of inconsistency for religious critics.

Second, my analysis of the ownership objection demonstrates that it ultimately carries more of a symbolic function for religious critics than a literal one. Although more philosophical work on the nature of intellectual property remains to be done, to the extent that patents do not entail full ownership, the religious argument on that score is off the mark. In addition, subsequent discussion among theologians regarding the sovereignty claim about human beings being pre-owned by God has also shown this objection to be theologically underdeveloped and still quite contestable. God's "ownership" of human beings and all creation cannot be strictly analogized to human ownership. To recall Cole-Turner's argument, God does not own all things in the same exclusive sense that human ownership entails.

Objections to patenting related to commodification in the narrow sense of the term are likewise problematic. Commodification in the narrow sense requires an exchange of goods or services for money. Since nothing can be bought or sold unless it is first owned, patented genes do not fall within this narrow definition. Unless the narrow understanding can be more compellingly applied to patenting, the religious objections in the literal sense are insufficient to warrant change in the patent system.

If, however, the term ownership does serve as a placeholder for a family of moral and religious concerns as I have suggested, and if commodification is understood in the broader sense suggested by Radin, the religious objections are not ethically vacuous. What these objections demonstrate is that patenting represents a further encroachment of market valuation to an area in which the issues at stake are how we value life forms generally, and our human selves especially. Given the growing "geneticization" of life—that trend toward the redescription of human life and experience in terms of genetic "determinants"—and the power of genetic essentialism within culture, ownership and commodification concerns are worthy of special attention. While human beings and other life forms may not be reducible to their genes, genetic science is teaching us more and more how genes are integrally related to individual identity. The closer and more extensive the connection we make between gene and self, the greater our interest should be in how we think about and value genetic material.

Within the prevailing economic and liberal political systems of the Western world—increasingly united by international trade agreements—little can be done to prevent virtually all aspects of life from succumbing to some degree of market rhetoric and valuation. Perhaps, then, the most important and morally significant role of religious traditions in this and future debates about biotechnology can be the way in which they function prophetically to preserve at least "incomplete commodification" in relation to genes and biological material. That is, the ways they can help to maintain descriptions of these materials and patentable life forms that preserve features worthy of moral attention—such as the way that certain genes are integral to identity, or that genes and life forms are parts of complex ecosystems. Although the secular world may not adopt the alternative religious world views or conceptual schemes within which religious critics understand DNA and gene patenting, the presence of alternatives that preserve important religious and secular values within public discourse is crucial to a social morality rich enough to inhibit the sorts of abuses that market reductionism may promote. Similar conclusions apply to the religious objections related to gene patenting as promoting philosophical materialism and social injustice.

These conclusions are themselves problematic, however. It might be argued, for example, that a debate which turns primarily on "semantics" or mere discourse is ethically insignificant and not worth attending to once the dust settles and the public policies have been established. Patenting of genetic and other biological material is, after all, the law of the land, save for some minor issues to be worked out regarding the patentability of certain raw genetic sequences without known function.

I have already suggested the general importance of preserving a richness of description regarding genetic materials. To push that point a bit further, I turn again to Radin. She makes three relevant suggestions as to why the encroachment of market discourse matters. First, market rhetoric "might lead less-than-perfect practitioners to wrong answers in sensitive cases."[69] A discourse that reduces policy decisions solely to matters of marketplace considerations has difficulties accommodating other values that may be necessary for sound, ethical decisions in difficult cases. For example, considering agricultural crops and their genetic structures merely as commodities may inhibit ecological and cultural considerations when making policy regarding the desirability of genetically engineered crops. Similarly, if our discourse about human genetic materials becomes too commodified, the loss of broader understandings may skew a range of difficult policy and ethical decisions regarding our genetic identities. The problem with the religious objections, however, is that patenting plays too small a role in our public discourse for concerns about market rhetoric to pull much weight against the benefits patenting allows.

Radin's second argument for why discourse matters relates to the effect how we talk may have on personhood:

> Systematically conceiving of personal attributes as fungible objects is threatening to personhood because it detaches from the person that which is integral to the person. . . . Moreover, if my bodily integrity is an integral personal attribute, not a detachable object, then hypothetically valuing my bodily integrity in terms of money is not far removed from valuing me in terms of money.[70]

As Brody's analysis illustrates, this argument may provide something of a wedge against the move toward patenting an entire genetically engineered human embryo, for instance. But equating the patenting of gene fragments with personhood or bodily integrity would be an extreme form of genetic reductionism. (Cloning raises this issue even more directly, of course.)

A third reason discourse matters is that "there is no such thing as two radically different normative discourses reaching the 'same' result."[71] We experience our world largely as we construct it. As Radin suggests, the rhetorics we use to describe the world and our experience are intimately related to and reflective of our broader commitments to human flourishing. Reductionist descriptions of human identity of any kind thus entail certain moral dangers for how we construct our views of ourselves and our ethical responsibilities to each other.

I believe the fallout of these arguments for the gene patenting debate lies in reinforcing the importance of walking a fine line between two forms of reductionism. On the one hand, I have argued the importance of avoiding the market and materialist rhetoric enabled by viewing DNA as merely chemical. Biotechnology is in fact engaging in a serious endeavor by placing the hand of human manipulation on the "building blocks" that are integral to identity, guided only by a human wisdom torn between the promotion of well-being and the pursuit of profit. On the other hand, it seems important to avoid a reductionism that places too much of the sanctity of life and species or individual identity within the genes themselves. Such a view is not only inaccurate, it may unnecessarily raise obstacles to the ethical pursuits of biotechnology and create unhelpful misunderstanding between biotechnology and all those concerned with the direction and implications of its development.

Religious traditions and those in biotechnology and industry would be best served by recognizing and striving to sustain the rich variety of ways in which we value genetic materials and organisms. Noneconomic and economic modes of description and valuing, for example, can coexist—something largely overlooked by religious critics. By not only recognizing the values and world views that motivate others, but also trying to understand, address, and, where possible, accommodate the significant values they represent, representatives of competing perspectives can constructively engage each other even if their values remain in some tension.

Practically speaking, whatever its shortcomings, the utility of the current patent system for promoting the ethical goals of the biotechnology industry is undeniable. Certain limited forms of commodification of genetic material and other life forms may be a price worth paying for the morally imperative goods that biotechnology can offer, such as health and environmental conservation. Many religionists support this view. And as Brody has pointed out, worries about the commodification of genes may be a luxury only wealthier, high-technology countries can afford; certain kinds of commodification can even be a good thing.[72]

One of the reasons for religious opposition to gene patenting, however, lies in the belief that there are feasible alternatives to promote those goals without the moral costs entailed by patenting itself. Rabbi Saperstein's remarks at the joint appeal make this point strongly:

> I am not here today to deny the immeasurable benefits of genetic engineering. . . . However, the biotech industry would be able to continue discovering these marvels of science without the patenting process. Numerous products have already been created, manufactured, and marketed without patents. The only undeniable benefit of issuing patents for genetically engineered life forms is the monopolization of profits by the invested industries.[73]

Furthermore, the acceptance of process patents—patents on the processes of invention rather than their objects—by religious critics indicates that their objections are not simply a cover for broader objections to the technology itself or its potential abuse. Thus, if patents remain the only possibility for promoting the ethically defensible goals of biotechnology—and the jury still seems out on this—the efforts of the industry should be focused on making this case, rather than simply reiterating the definition of patents.

Further Dialogue: Specific Recommendations

While the patenting of genes and other biological materials is now firmly set by legal precedent and well entrenched in practice, there remain unresolved issues and uncertainties on the horizon. The patentability of raw DNA sequence data with no known function (at least not at the time of patent application) has been a source of confusion and ongoing debate. Perhaps more relevant for religious communities will be the possible patentability of certain genetically engineered organisms. The cloning of genetically engineered plants and animals represents another front on which the morality of some patents may come into question, particularly if those organisms are made vulnerable to suffering or purposes potentially detrimental to ecosystems. Such cases will likely raise familiar concerns of commodification and ownership, but also bring additional issues to the foreground, such as the integrity of species identity.

From the discussions that have occurred thus far, both in the literature as well as in such forums as the Dialogue Program between Science and Religion of the American Association for the Advancement of Science and The Hastings Center's Values and Biotechnology Program, I believe certain recommendations follow.

Dialogue would benefit from greater attention to and mutual understanding of positions on the following substantive issues.

The meaning of DNA. Parties to the dialogue need to have well-developed and clear positions on how they understand genes and DNA. This will require more theological work within religious traditions and a more open acknowledgment by the industry of the various ways DNA is valued, even and especially within industry itself. Finally, the interlocutors must ask what is at stake ethically and socially with various meanings of DNA.

The question of ownership. The term ownership has been used in different ways in this debate to suit different rhetorical purposes. The dialogue would benefit from more direct attention to legal and philosophical conceptions of ownership in relation to patenting. Theologically, more work is needed regarding how we might better understand "God's ownership," and what implications that would have for human ownership.

How patenting entails commodification. The issue of commodification captures a range of concerns related to the development of biotechnology. The case of patenting offers an opportunity to explore them further, with special attention to the meanings of commodification, the implications of it for the future direction of biotechnology, and in which cases commodification might be morally problematic, or morally necessary, or even morally imperative. In addition, much more critical work could be done to help foster shared considerations of the morality of patenting for certain future technologies.

Ethical dimensions of this debate should be considered in reference to application of the patent law in certain contestable circumstances, in reference to both current and possible future technologies.

Certain technologies or potentially patentable materials may raise values questions more directly than the general patenting of genes with known function. Examples include DNA sequences data; genetically engineered organisms that suffer or whose genetic identity is substantially changed; genetically engineered human embryos for research; cloning; and others. Greater clarity on the value dimensions of patenting generally, along with proactive consideration of future developments would lead to more constructive dialogue and help avert controversy.

More attention is needed to how the United States patent system might recover and accommodate some consideration of the public good and broad public morality.

There is some consensus among parties to the patenting debate that the U.S. Patent and Trademark Office may not be the best place for moral considerations to enter into judgment and control of biotechnology or any other technology. And as Leon Kass has argued, the courts are not best suited to take on the job of "brakeman."[74] It may be useful, however, to explore the values implied by how patent applications are evaluated, interpretations of what constitutes patentable subject matter, and what review mechanisms might be proposed for potentially objectionable patents.

More consideration should be given to alternatives to patenting of genes and other biological materials.

Given the questions that still remain—ranging from the economics of patenting, to its effects on research, to its moral compromises—a fuller exploration of alternatives to or modifications of the patent system would be useful for promoting the important goals of biotechnology and overcoming public controversy, especially in future cases.

Extending the Dialogue between Religion and Biotechnology: General Recommendations

Perhaps the most valuable consequence of the debate stirred up by the religious leaders in the 1995 joint appeal has been the renewed attention to values that religious traditions represent and the dialogue that has resulted, not only among theologians and religious leaders, but especially between religious leaders and representatives of the biotechnology industry. The experience of dialogue on the gene patenting issue should be seen as a beginning of conversations on many issues to come. The patenting debate began to reveal some of the values and religious issues that biotechnology in general will continue to raise: the relation of DNA to identity, the concerns with inappropriate commodification and corporate control, and the positive goals of health and well-being.

The patenting debate also helped move future discussions to a richer level, not merely by revealing the complexity of the issues involved, but also by breaking down simple dichotomies of religion versus science/industry. For as I have stated, there is not only disagreement among religious believers on many of these issues, but there are disagreements among those in science and industry as well. Furthermore, it is often overlooked that scientists often belong to religious traditions.

As new issues break into the public attention—as cloning did without warning—an ongoing dialogue will be especially important if knee-jerk responses are to be avoided and if responsible policies that take account of a diversity of values are to be developed. Thus the gene patenting debate suggests several general recommendations for broader future dialogue within and between religion and biotechnology:

Religious communities and theologians need to identify and research the theological dimensions of new genetic technologies.

With a few exceptions, religious groups and theologians are currently not giving enough attention to the challenges raised by emerging genetic technologies. As a result, they are often ill prepared to face new developments and offer meaningful participation in public dialogue or provide for the education of their own communities. Lacking sufficient research and discussion, their public arguments are vague and may fail to draw intelligible connections between their public conclusions and the reasoning that led to them. Without such connections, use of religious language for authority and justification becomes empty and public dialogue unproductive.

Leaders of the biotechnology industry should further educate themselves about the range of values questions raised by the products they develop and the processes they employ, and resist the temptation to approach moral and religious issues merely as marketing or communications problems.

The patenting debate illustrates the extent to which issues run deeper than the moral questions acknowledged by the industry thus far. Characterizing moral issues in biotechnology as marketing or communications problems lends itself to a strategy of "consumer education," in which it is assumed that greater education about the science and products of biotechnology will suffice to alleviate possible controversies. While such education raises general acceptance of biotechnology, it ultimately fails adequately to address or accommodate what may be valid moral/religious concerns and may lead to greater miscommunication and misunderstandings down the line. The industry should take steps to support and participate in academic research and dialogue groups that promote mutual education and understanding (as it has begun to do).

Religious traditions should not be faulted for sounding alarms of caution regarding certain developments in biotechnology.

It is integral to the mission of many religious traditions to question attempts by human beings to usurp power in the manipulation of life. Religious traditions can thus be seen as playing an important social role as a monitor of technological developments that may threaten significant social, moral, or religious values. Even when a pluralistic society may find compelling policy reasons for rejecting the arguments of religious groups, the society is nonetheless served by the presence of a "prophetic minority" that can enrich public moral discourse and witness to other important values.

Religious traditions should take care not to react to biotechnological developments in ways that diminish the potential power of their voice in public debates about biotechnology.

Although working together with Jeremy Rifkin may have served the purpose of getting the issue on the front page of the *New York Times*, as one coalition leader put it, alliances with groups that oppose biotechnology generally may both poison the atmosphere for dialogue as well as create opportunities for misunderstanding regarding the substance of the religious and moral concerns being raised.

In addition, it is also important for religionists to enter into dialogue with an adequate grasp of the scientific, legal, and economic dimensions of the issues at stake.

Parties to dialogue need to take great care with the "idioms" they use in communication with each other.

All parties to future discussion should recognize that the idioms of communication they employ represent particular modes of understanding reality that all people may not share—even on what seem to be points of indisputable fact.

Those speaking out of religious traditions have perhaps the more difficult task of communication, for those traditions typically employ different modes of discourse in various settings, which can be characterized by how they utilize largely prophetic, ethical, narrative, and policy idioms.[75] Careful selection of the appropriate mode of discourse is necessary to keep communication clear and intelligible to target audiences. Special care should be taken by religious traditions when "translating" religious and especially prophetic discourse into policy terms. For example, in the gene patenting debate, "ownership" in reference to DNA was used symbolically by religious leaders to serve a prophetic function and was thus largely misunderstood by those in industry, who used the term in a different sense. In addition, when religious groups are not careful to target their communication appropriately to specific audiences, they contribute to an unhelpful mixing of types of religious and secular idioms.

Those representing nonreligious perspectives have also employed a variety of idioms, for example, describing DNA in terms ranging from "the holy grail" (in public relations and fund-raising contexts) to "merely chemical" (in patenting contexts). They, therefore, also have an obligation both to represent the partiality of their own idioms and frames of reference, and also to press for common ways of communicating with those whose perspectives may be different.

Expressions of concern from religious groups should be explored for the values they express—whether common or distinctive.

Despite the use of religious language and justification, many religious concerns find similar voices among other secular groups. The gene patenting controversy demonstrates that although religious positions were often not well articulated, they nonetheless bore witness to issues such as commodification, deliberation about which can enrich further moral and policy considerations. Concerns raised by religious groups often find parallel articulations within secular groups. Areas of overlap would be especially fruitful to explore for shared values and modes of expression.

Greater attention to the ethical implications of the commercialization of biotechnology is fundamental to many future dialogues at the intersection of religion and biotechnology.

Beyond challenges to what we understand the meaning of DNA to be, the increasing commercialization of genetic technologies will introduce many challenges to human values and issues of human and other species' identities. Religious communities are not sufficiently prepared to offer understanding and guidance on such matters from their own traditions. The biotechnology industry will also need to increase its attention to such matters and enter into constructive and sincere relationships with those who may offer guidance—including patient groups, religious organizations, ethics research centers, and private consultants. Failing that, collaboration and mutual trust will diminish.

Greater mutual trust may result from focus on shared values—such as improved health and environmental outcomes—and the ways in which commercialization and commodification in biotechnology can be compatible with other ways of valuing biological materials.

Industry, religious groups, and third-party research groups should take initiative to identify and discuss developments on the horizon of biotechnology that may raise new value questions.

When possible, proactive efforts should be taken to engage in education and dialogue on future possibilities in biotechnology. This would help those outside the industry learn what issues they might be thinking about and obviate the need for critics to resort to press conferences after the fact. The question of germ-line gene therapy is an example of an issue that will likely draw attention in the future.

It is clear that the future of biotechnology will bring many occasions for persons of all religious and moral traditions to feel challenged regarding fundamental ethical questions. The capacity adequately to address these challenges will depend on the richness of the moral resources available for public dialogue, and the willingness of persons to appreciate and understand them. For this reason, the public dialogue, and ultimately our policies on biotechnology, will only be diminished if we disallow distinctive contributions from the unique traditions that not everyone shares. The religious voices in the gene patenting debate were important not because their objections to patenting were on or off target, but because they showed the rest of us the value of main-taining a morally rich language for thinking about genetics generally, and the need for constructive dialogue on matters of values. Mutual education and informed conversation about plural perspectives on values and biotechnology are the best means for discovering shared and diverging values and ultimately making wise decisions for biotechnology's future.

NOTES

1. For example, many presentations at the conference "Resisting the Commercialization of Our Genes" sponsored by The Council for Responsible Genetics (26 October 1996) contained rhetoric that paralleled religious concerns.

2. "Statement of the Biotechnology Industry Organization Regarding Bioethics Issues," submitted to the Senate Labor and Human Resources Committee, 25 July 1996, p. 14.

3. Richard Stone, "Religious Leaders Oppose Patenting Genes and Animals," *Science* 268 (26 May 1995): 1126.

4. U.S. Congress, Office of Technology Assessment, *New Developments in Biotechnology: Patenting Life-Special Report*, OTA-BA-370 (Washington, D.C.: U.S. Government Printing Office, 1989), p. 30.

5. For discussions of the views of the churches, see Ronald Cole-Turner, *The New Genesis: Theology and the Genetic Revolution* (Louisville, Ky.: Westminster/John Knox Press, 1995), pp. 70–78; Mark Ellingsen, *The Cutting Edge: How the Churches Speak on Social Issues* (Grand Rapids, Mich.: Wm. B. Eerdmans Publishing Co., 1993), pp. 103–10, and 299–304.

6. Stone, "Religious Leaders Oppose Patenting Genes and Animals," p. 1126.

7. "United Methodist Church Genetic Science Task Force Report to the 1992 General Conference," pp. 113–23, at 121.

8. For example, "Today's Debate: Genetics versus Religion," *USA Today*, 19 May 1995; "Thou Shalt Not Patent! Religion: A Clergy Coalition Battles Biotechnology," *Newsweek*, 29 May 1995.

9. Mark Sagoff, "Patenting Genetic Resources: A Survey of Normative and Conceptual Issues," in *Perspectives on Genetic Patenting: Religion, Science, and Industry in Dialogue*, ed. Audrey R. Chapman (Washington, D.C.: American Association for the Advancement of Science, 1999), pp. 245–68.

10. Rebecca S. Eisenberg, "Structure and Function in Gene Patenting," *Nature Genetics* 15 (1997): 125–30, at 125.

11. Dorothy Nelkin and Susan Lindee, *The DNA Mystique: The Gene as a Cultural Icon* (New York: W. H. Freeman and Company, 1995), p. 39.

12. Nelkin and Lindee, *The DNA Mystique*, p. 140. It is worth noting, however, that the characteristics of the soul as immortal and independent of the body are of Greek origin and not consistent with most Christian theology, despite popular beliefs to the contrary. Nelkin and Lindee's description is therefore misleading on this point.

13. Nelkin and Lindee, *The DNA Mystique*, p. 41.

14. Nelkin and Lindee, *The DNA Mystique*, pp. 41–42.

15. Kate H. Murashige, "Intellectual Property and Genetic Testing," in *The Genetic Frontier: Ethics, Law, and Policy*, ed. Mark S. Frankel and Albert

Teich (Washington, D.C.: American Association for the Advancement of Science, 1994), pp. 181–98, at p. 184.

16. Leon R. Kass, *Toward a More Natural Science: Biology and Human Affairs* (New York: The Free Press, 1985), pp. 128–53.

17. Kass, *Toward a More Natural Science*, p. 135.

18. Kass also discusses the implicit tensions within patent law, such as between "self-interest and common good, monopoly and liberty, the ownership of ideas and the shareability or publicity of speech and thought." See Kass, *Toward a More Natural Science*, p. 136.

19. E. Richard Gold, *Body Parts: Property Rights and the Ownership of Human Biological Materials* (Washington, D.C.: Georgetown University Press, 1996), p. 67.

20. Gold, *Body Parts*, pp. 80–85.

21. Eisenberg, "Structure and Function in Gene Patenting," p. 125. According to Eisenberg, patentability also extends to recombinant vectors and host cells that include DNA sequences.

22. Cathleen Kaveny, "Religious Values, Cultural Symbols, and the Law." Paper presented to the Religion and Biotechnology Project at The Hastings Center, Briarcliff Manor, N.Y., 18 April 1997.

23. Kaveny, "Religious Values, Cultural Symbols, and the Law."

24. Biotechnology Industry Organization, "Statement of the Biotechnology Industry Organization Regarding Bioethics Issues," 25 July 1996, p. 14.

25. George Poste, "The Case for Genomic Patenting," *Nature* 378 (1995): 534–536, at 534.

26. Poste, "The Case for Genomic Patenting," p. 535.

27. Biotechnology Industry Organization, "Statement of the Biotechnology Industry Organization Regarding Bioethics Issues," p. 15.

28. George Poste, David Roberts, and Simon Gentry, "Patents, Ethics, and Improving Healthcare," *Bulletin of Medical Ethics* 124 (January 1997): 29–31, at 31.

29. Pharmaceutical Research and Manufacturers of America, news release, 18 May 1995.

30. Poste et al., "Patents, Ethics, and Improving Healthcare," p. 30.

31. Michele Svatos, "Biotechnology and the Utilitarian Argument for Patents," *Social Philosophy and Policy* 13, no. 2 (1996): 113–44.

32. James Mason and Michael Drummond, "Biotechnology: A Special Case for Health Technology Assessment?" *Health Policy* 41, no. 1 (1997): 73–81.

33. Statement of Dr. Richard D. Land to the National Press Club, 18 May 1995.

34. Richard D. Land and C. Ben Mitchell, "Patenting Life: No," *First Things* 63 (May 1996): 20–22, at 21; Rabbi David Saperstein's statements also imply an ownership argument against patenting: "On this our faith is clear: we do not own this world we inhabit; rather, we are its stewards—God, its

Creator, is its only true owner." See David Saperstein, "Press Release," 18 May 1995, of the Religious Action Center of Reform Judaism.

35. Judith Andre, "Blocked Exchanges: A Taxonomy," *Ethics* 103, no. 1 (1992): 29–47, at 32.

36. In fact, philosopher Baruch Brody, who is studying the nature of intellectual property, argues that critics of patenting are not mistaken in applying the term ownership to the intellectual property rights applied to biological materials. Personal conversation, 13 March 1997.

37. Indeed, it is remarkable the extent to which the term ownership is used even by those in biotechnology and patent law. Patent attorney Kate H. Murashige's use of "ownership" in quotation marks seems to indicate that the term may be the closest we have to convey meaning even if, in legal terms, it is not technically the most accurate. An example of such a use of the term in literature on the topic would be S. M. Thomas et al., "Ownership of the Human Genome," *Nature* 380 (4 April 1996): 387–88.

38. Land and Mitchell, "Patenting Life: No," p. 20.

39. Land and Mitchell, "Patenting Life: No," p. 21.

40. Kenneth L. Carder, Statement on Patenting of Genes, 18 May 1995, p. 1.

41. Audrey R. Chapman, "Human Genetic Patenting: Ethical and Theological Issues," Paper presented at the annual meeting of the Society of Christian Ethics, Cincinnati, Ohio, 11 January 1997, p. 14.

42. Chapman, "Human Genetic Patenting," p. 14.

43. Andre, "Blocked Exchanges," p. 33.

44. Andre, "Blocked Exchanges," p. 33.

45. Ronald Cole-Turner, "The Theological Status of DNA: A Contribution to the Debate over Gene Patenting," in *Perspectives on Genetic Patenting: Religion, Science, and Industry in Dialogue*, ed. Audrey R. Chapman (Washington, D.C.: American Association for the Advancement of Science, 1999), pp. 149–66, at 152.

46. Andre, "Blocked Exchanges," p. 34.

47. Land and Mitchell, "Patenting Life: No," p. 22; see Kass, *Toward a More Natural Science*, p. 151.

48. Carder, Statement on Patenting of Genes, p. 1.

49. Margaret Jane Radin, *Contested Commodities* (Cambridge, Mass.: Harvard University Press, 1996), p. 12.

50. Radin, *Contested Commodities*, p. 13.

51. Radin, *Contested Commodities*, p. 2.

52. Radin, *Contested Commodities*, p. 2.

53. Radin, *Contested Commodities*, p. 8.

54. Radin, *Contested Commodities*, p. 13.

55. Land and Mitchell, "Patenting Life: No," p. 22.

56. Richard D. Land, Statement of Dr. Richard D. Land, 18 May 1995, p. 3.

57. Saperstein, Press Release, p. 1.

58. Radin, *Contested Commodities*, pp. 102–14. Complete and literal commodification would involve "(1) exchanges of things in the world (2) for money, (3) in the social context of markets, and (4) in conjunction with four indicia of commodification in conceptualization. Those four conceptual indicia characterize complete commodification in rhetoric. They are (i) objectification, (ii) fungibility, (iii) commensurability, and (iv) money equivalence." See Radin, *Contested Commodities*, p. 118.

59. Ted Peters, "Should We Patent God's Creation?" *Dialogue* 35, no. 2 (1996): 117–32, at 123.

60. For an analysis of this topic, see Baruch A. Brody, "Protecting Human Dignity and the Patenting of Human Genes," in *Perspectives on Genetic Patenting: Religion, Science, and Industry in Dialogue*, ed. Audrey R. Chapman (Washington, D.C.: American Association for the Advancement of Science, 1999), pp. 111–26.

61. Brody, "Protecting Human Dignity," p. 11.

62. Brody, "Protecting Human Dignity," p. 11. See also M. Nelson, "The Morality of the Market in Transplant Organs," *Public Affairs Quarterly* 5 (1991): 63–79.

63. Commission of the European Communities, "Amended Proposal for a Council Directive on the Legal Protection of Biotechnological Inventions," COM (92) 589 final-SYN 159 (Brussels: 16 December 1992).

64. Land and Mitchell, "Patenting Life: No," p. 21.

65. Carder, Statement on Patenting of Genes, p. 1.

66. Kass, Toward a More Natural Science, pp. 149–50.

67. See Beth Burrows, "Second Thoughts about U.S. Patent #4,438,032," *Bulletin of Medical Ethics* 124 (January 1997): 11–14.

68. Chapman, "Human Genetic Patenting," p. 6.

69. Radin, *Contested Commodities*, pp. 84–85.

70. Radin, *Contested Commodities*, p. 88.

71. Radin, *Contested Commodities*, p. 84.

72. This point was made by Baruch Brody at a meeting of the Religion and Biotechnology Project at The Hastings Center, Briarcliff Manor, N.Y., 18 June 1996.

73. Saperstein, Press Release, p. 2.

74. Kass, Toward a More Natural Science, p. 143.

75. James F. Gustafson, "Moral Discourse about Medicine: A Variety of Forms," *The Journal of Medicine and Philosophy* 15, no. 2 (1990): 125–42.

AUDREY R. CHAPMAN

Religious Perspectives on Biotechnology[1]

In June 1980, leaders of three major religious communities—Protestant, Catholic, and Jewish—took the unusual step of writing to the U.S. president to express their concerns about a recent scientific development. The letter from the general secretaries of the National Council of Churches, the United States Catholic Conference, and the Synagogue Council of America to President Jimmy Carter warned of the perils that genetic engineering posed to humanity:

> We are rapidly moving into a new era of fundamental danger triggered by the rapid growth of genetic engineering. Albeit, there may be opportunity for doing good; the very term suggests the danger. Who shall determine how human good is best served when new life forms are being engineered? Who shall control genetic experimentation and its results which could have untold implications for human survival? Who will benefit and who will bear any adverse consequences, directly or indirectly?[2]

The letter went on to state that these were not ordinary issues. "These are moral, ethical, and religious questions. They deal with the fundamental nature of human life and the dignity and worth of the individual human being."[3] The general secretaries requested that the president convene a group to consider these matters and advise the government. In turn, they pledged their own efforts: "The religious community must and will address these fundamental questions in a more urgent and organized way."[4] And in the past two decades members of the religious community, on both a corporate and individual level, have sought to raise and address these questions in a variety of ways.

I have just completed a review and evaluation of the literature contributed by religious ethicists on genetics, cloning, genetic patenting, and human nature in light of genetic discoveries. The analysis appears in a book titled *Unprecedented Choices: Religious Ethics at the Frontiers of*

Genetic Science.[5] The study grew out of my belief that religious thought can potentially make a significant contribution both to the religious community and to broader societal efforts to grapple with the choices and dilemmas arising from the genetics revolution. Religious perspectives on genetics can offer broad frameworks of understanding and the moral vision so necessary to deal with these complex issues. Theologians and ethicists can draw on centuries, indeed millennia, of reflections about the nature of the person, human relationships, and social responsibilities. In contrast with the radical individualism so prevalent in our society, most religious traditions have a conception of human beings as basically social and interdependent beings and a commitment to the common good. Religious thinkers also tend to interpret human life and destiny in more inclusive contexts of meaning and purpose than secular philosophers and ethicists.

Nevertheless, the emphasis should be on the word "potentially" in the affirmation that religious ethics are relevant to the task of shaping a moral response to the impact and implications of biotechnology. The genetic revolution offers both a challenge and an opportunity to religious communities: a challenge to apply religious values and frameworks to new and unprecedented issues, and an opportunity to help interpret and illuminate significant ethical choices before members and the wider society. Religious thinkers have to surmount various methodological issues and other liabilities before they can shape a meaningful and effective moral response to the genetics revolution. The lack of deep knowledge about genetic science is not the only obstacle. Some commentators assume that religious communities or thinkers have positions based on their heritage that they can readily apply to biotechnology, but clearly that is not the case. As one theologian commentated about the discussion of cloning, "You can't just take a (religious) tradition that has been worked out in centuries of cultural shift and apply it like a cookbook to a new discovery."[6] Written within the context of prescientific societies, the foundational texts of most religious communities do not speak directly to the ethical dilemmas raised by biotechnology. Moreover, philosophical, ethical, and theological concepts that were relevant to the intellectual milieu of past centuries do not easily illuminate the interpretation and analysis of contemporary science. In addition, religious principles and norms tend to be formulated in such an abstract manner that they require "operationalization" to become sufficiently concrete to be pertinent to empirical scientific developments. One of the central themes of *Unprecedented Choices* is that traditional ethical and theological building blocks need to be informed by, and in some cases revised through, a dialogue with science.

This chapter will draw on some of the observations in my book. It will begin by providing an overview of this literature. It will then analyze the type of ethic contributed by religious thinkers, with separate sections on ethical/prophetic discourse and public theology. The third section will deal with similarities and differences in religious and secular ethics on biotechnology. The final section will evaluate the contribution of these works.

Overview of the Literature

During the past twenty years, various ecumenical bodies and many of the major Christian communions in the United States have formulated policy statements on issues related to genetics and commissioned pastoral and study resources for their members. The World Council of Churches organized its first consultation on genetics as early as 1973, focusing on issues of genetic counseling,[7] and then dealt with genetics at their 1979 World Conference on Faith, Science and the Future at the Massachusetts Institute of Technology. Following that conference, the World Council of Churches convened a working group that prepared the 1982 report *Manipulating Life: Ethical Issues in Genetic Engineering.*[8] In 1989, the World Council of Churches Subunit on Church and Society issued another report titled *Biotechnology: Its Challenges to the Churches and the World.*[9] In 1980, the National Council of the Churches of Christ in the U.S.A. organized its first task force, whose membership included both scientists and several theological ethicists, which spent three years preparing a report titled *Human Life and the New Genetics.*[10] Subsequently, the National Council of the Churches appointed another panel, which in 1984 produced a book titled *Genetic Engineering: Social and Ethical Consequences.*[11] Then in 1986, the Governing Board formally adopted a statement entitled "Genetic Science for Human Benefit" that was published as a sixteen-page pamphlet.[12]

Of the documents within the Roman Catholic tradition with implications for genetics and genetic engineering, *Instruction on Respect for Human Life in its Origin and on the Dignity of Life (Donum Vitae),*[13] issued by the Congregation for the Doctrine of the Faith in 1987, is perhaps the most significant, and unlike most of the ecumenical Protestant documents listed above, it has the status of a magisterial statement seeking to clarify and restate official teaching. Other resources setting forth a Catholic perspective include an address Pope John Paul II made on medical ethics and genetic manipulation in 1983 to participants in the World Medical Association convention that was reproduced in *Origins*, the U.S. national Catholic documentary service.[14] In 1990, the Catholic Health Association of the United States issued *Human Genetics: Ethical Issues in Genetic Testing, Counseling, and Therapy*,[15] developed by an interdisciplinary research group to serve as a resource for ethical consultation and decision making. A working party of the British Catholic Bishops' Joint Committee on Bioethical Issues undertook a four-year study of human genetics and produced a resource that considers both somatic (nonheritable) and germ-line (heritable) interventions.[16]

Eight major North American Protestant denominations have addressed genetics issues in some form, and at least one European communion, the Church of Scotland, has also done so. As might be anticipated, these denominational documents are very different in focus, purpose, and emphasis, as well as the process by which they were drafted. Of the group, seven—the United Methodist Church, the United Church of Christ, the Episcopal Church, the Presbyterian Church (U.S.A.), the Reformed Church in America, the Evangelical Lutheran Church in America, and the Southern Baptist Convention—have drafted reports, policy statements, or study resources on genetic science, genetic engineering, or procreational ethics, and an eighth, the United Church of Canada, has prepared a brief for submission to the (Canadian) Royal Commission on New Reproductive Technologies. Responding to the revolution in biomedical technology, in 1983 the newly reunited Presbyterian Church General Assembly devoted a section of its report on biomedical issues, titled "The Covenant of Life and the Caring Community," to "Genetic Choices and the Ethics of Domination,"[17] and in 1990, the Presbyterian General Assembly adopted a second resolution.[18] After a process that involved development of a provisional study by its Commission on Christian Action, congregational study, and a series of consultations, the General Synod of the Reformed Church approved a statement on genetic engineering in 1988.[19] In 1989, the Seventeenth General Synod of the United Church of Christ voted on a pronouncement, the "Church and Genetic Engineering,"[20] and a related resolution, "The Church and Reproductive Technologies."[21] Two years later, the 70th General Conference of the Episcopal Church passed a resolution providing guidelines in the area of genetic engineering. A report of the United Methodist Church Genetic Science Task Force was adopted by the 1992 General Conference under the title "New Developments in Genetic Science."[22] Somewhat ironically, the text that arguably is reasoned most clearly from a theological foundation is not a denominational resolution but a brief to the Royal Commission on New Reproductive Technologies prepared on behalf of The United Church of Canada by their Division of Mission.[23]

Several "second-generation" studies of human genetics and genetic engineering by expert study groups set up by various denominations are underway or in some cases completed. In 1998, the Office of Theology and Worship of the Congregational Ministries Division of the Presbyterian Church (U.S.A.) published a collection of essays titled *In Whose Image? Faith, Science, and the New Genetics* intended for personal and group study. The volume focuses on the "challenge that contemporary developments in the biological sciences pose to the church's theology, and especially, to the church's understanding of what it means to be human before God."[24] The Committee on Medical Ethics of the Episcopal Diocese of Washington also published a work in 1998 titled *Wrestling with the Future: Our Genes and Our Choices*, which offers an overview of issues related to prenatal and adult genetic testing.[25] Likewise, *Genetic Testing and Screening: Critical Engagement at the Intersection of Faith and Science*, sponsored by the Division for Church in Society of the Evangelical Lutheran Church in America, is an edited volume, with study questions following each chapter.[26] In contrast with the Episcopal resource on genetic testing, which has an emphasis on explaining the options and their implications, *Genetic Testing and Screening* places these issues within a more substantive theological and ethical framework. A resource on the ethics of genetic engineering in nonhuman species, developed by a working group of the Society, Religion and Technology Project of the Church of Scotland, was also published in 1998.[27] At the time of this writing, the United Church of Christ is completing work on a collection of essays based on a series of cases, each dealing with a different dimension of the moral dilemmas that genetics raises.

These "second-generation" works often have more in common with the writings of individual scholars than the initial round of denomination-commissioned and -drafted resources. Perhaps that should not be surprising given the composition of the working groups, many of whom are the same people. In contrast with the earlier denominational efforts that sought primarily to establish baseline policies, these are efforts to develop serious, in-depth treatments of the way that genetics intersects with and challenges traditional theological understandings. The focus on the ethical and theological issues genetic testing raises reflects the realization that "It is largely through genetic testing and screening that the nonspecialist will personally confront the personal, social, theological, and pastoral dilemmas that attend genetic developments."[28] Although these resources were prepared under the sponsorship of particular denominations, they are only loosely linked with historical confessions and earlier policy positions.

There is also a growing ethical and theological literature on genetics by moral theologians in the form of individually authored book-length studies, articles, edited collections of articles, and chapters of broader works. Yet, despite the recognition of the significance of the discoveries in the field of genetics, fewer than a dozen book-length studies written by religious thinkers on this subject were published in the period between 1980 and 1998. There are also two edited collections on genetics based on contributions by religious ethicists.[29] Several of these works, particularly the individually authored book-length volumes, make a notable contribution toward identifying the moral and religious implications of genetic developments. Nevertheless, this literature is far from a comprehensive treatment of the ethical issues that genetic advances raise.

To briefly overview the major book-length works, in 1993 the United Church of Christ theologian Ronald Cole-Turner published *The New Genesis: Theology and the Genetic Revolution*. This relatively brief work (109 pages) provides a useful introduction to genetics and some of the theological issues the genetic revolution raises. *The New Genesis* considers the difference between traditional agricultural breeding methods and genetic engineering, the purpose of genetic engineering, and the initial response of the churches and individual theologians to developments in genetic research. Cole-Turner concludes with a series of theological affirmations that conceptualize genetic engineering as an extension of God's creating and redeeming activity. According to Cole-Turner, God works through both natural processes and human initiatives to achieve genetic changes. Nevertheless, he rejects the notion of humanity being imaged as God's co-creator in this process.[30]

Cole-Turner also coauthored a second book with Brent Waters, titled *Pastoral Genetics: Theology and Care at the Beginning of Life*,[31] whose primary intended audience is clergy attempting to counsel parishioners confronting the very difficult task of making moral decisions about procreation and abortion in an era of genetic testing. Far more than a "how-to" guide for clergy called on to provide guidance to parishioners, the book integrates an engaging case-study approach with an explanation of the scientific basis of genetic testing and a meaningful theological commentary. The three chapters connecting God with genetic processes, exploring the presence of God in pain, and considering human genetics in the light of the resurrection are particularly notable for their ability to take on very difficult, complex, and ambiguous issues and to illuminate without necessarily resolving them. Using a nondirective approach reminiscent of contemporary norms of pastoral counseling, their text informs pastoral genetics with sophisticated theological reflection without being prescriptive.

In 1994, J. Robert Nelson published a work titled *On the New Frontiers of Genetics and Religion*. The book recounts the presentations of participants prepared for two conferences organized by the Institute of Religion at the University of Texas in 1990 and 1992. In addition to Nelson's topical summaries of material dealt with in the two conferences, the book has excerpts from a few of the resources prepared for the conference and the text of a "Summary Reflection Statement" of the delegates at the second of the conferences. As might be expected, the book is a smorgasbord that bears many of the limitations of multiauthored volumes without the benefit of allowing the various voices speak for themselves. Because this publication is one of the few that seeks to incorporate a diversity of religious perspectives beyond the Christian community, it is particularly unfortunate that these were given so little space. The one exception is the essay on Judaism and genetics written by Barry Freundel, an Orthodox Jewish rabbi, as part of a working group report for the conference.[32]

Roger Shinn, who might be described as the doyenne of religious ethicists working on genetics issues, published a book in 1996 titled *The New Genetics: Challenges for Science, Faith, and Politics*.[33] In the work, Shinn argues that responsible decisions require both an understanding of the science and ethics. More specifically, he posits that public policies result from an interaction of three dynamic forces—human values and faiths, scientific information and concepts, and political activity.[34] One of the strengths of his treatment is to show the dialectic between the potential of genetic knowledge to heal and to distort the human. Because Shinn is writing for a secular rather than a religious audience, religion, to the extent it is dealt with at all, is considered more as a kind of ideological input into decision making rather than as a normative and conceptual context. The one exception is the chapter dealing with the modification of germ-line cells in which the issues are dealt with in a religious frame of reference.

Ted Peters' 1997 book, *Playing God? Genetic Determinism and Human Freedom*,[35] represents the first truly comprehensive and in-depth theological analysis of human genetics. Although religious thinkers had previously recognized that genetic knowledge raises issues for theological concepts and traditions, Peters is the first to systematically take on the challenge of exploring this knotty and complicated subject. The foreword, written by Francis Collins, Director of the National Center for Human Genome Research, describes the work as a "remarkable book,"[36] and this seems to be an apt characterization. As the subtitle indicates, the work examines the cultural and theological struggle between genetic determinism, the notion that our genes govern us like a puppeteer, and the hope that new genetic knowledge will increase the human freedom to control its own future and destiny. Peters, who is professor of systematic theology at Pacific Lutheran Theological Seminary and the Center for Theology and the Natural Science at the Graduate Theological Union in Berkeley, California, offers an eloquent criticism of the "gene myth" of genetic determinism and a defense of human moral freedom. The book argues that "responsibility includes building a better future through genetic science, a form of human creativity expressive of the image of God imparted by the divine to the human race."[37]

Jan Heller's *Human Genome Research and the Challenge of Contingent Future Persons*[38] investigates how genetic science is likely to affect future generations and explores the implications for evaluating the scientific advances associated with the Human Genome Project. Recognizing that future persons will bear the burdens and/or benefits of contemporary decisions about genetic science applications, particularly germ-line interventions that will be heritable, Heller seeks to find a philosophical and theological framework to utilize for moral deliberations.

Other topics related to genetic science have also received attention, albeit on a limited and intermittent basis. Within four months of the announcement of the successful cloning of a lamb from an adult cell, at least five official religious bodies issued statements opposing human cloning. Three of these were North American: the United Methodists, Southern Baptists, and the United Church of Christ. The Vatican and the Church of Scotland also made statements critical of the prospects of human cloning. Prompted at least in part by requests from the media, theologians and ethicists from a wide range of backgrounds also quickly contributed preliminary reflections on the ethical and religious meaning of human cloning. Thus far, only two books dealing with religious perspectives on cloning, both collections of short essays prepared by Ronald Cole-Turner, have been published.[39]

Concerns that genetic patenting demeans the dignity of life and/ or intrudes on divine prerogatives have led a very wide range of religious bodies, well beyond the Christian community, to criticize patents on life forms and genetic sequences. The best known of these is the 1995 "Joint Appeal Against Human and Animal Patenting," endorsed by leaders of some eighty religious faiths and denominations, including representatives of mainline Protestant denominations; Catholic, evangelical, charismatic, and Orthodox churches; and Jewish, Muslim, Buddhist, and Hindu communities. The controversy over this statement in turn engendered further commentary by various religious thinkers on the topic. Yet, despite the public attention and turmoil in the religious community, only two book-length studies have been published representing religious perspectives on the topic. The first is the proceedings of a workshop organized by the Institute for the Theological Encounter with Science and Technology,[40] and the other a collection of papers commissioned by a dialogue group operating under the aegis of the American Association for the Advancement of Science.[41]

Despite the early recognition that genetic research had significant implications for conceptions of human nature, work on updating traditional understandings of theological anthropology has been slow in coming, far slower than the ethical analysis generated by specific developments. Many of the ethicists writing on genetics during the past twenty years doubtlessly had some sense that genetic discoveries required reconsideration of traditional interpretations of human nature, but they deferred this project. This meant that evaluations of the implications of genetic discoveries tended to be based on interpretations of human nature that were at least partially outmoded by these and other scientific findings. In the 1990s, serious efforts were finally begun. Several were responding to the implied genetic essentialism and determinism of scientists, the media, and popular culture. Others can be considered to be evaluations of the claims of sociobiology. Still others, taking account of discoveries in the neurosciences as well as genetics, have reinterpreted the conception of the soul and the image of God. Overall, however, only a small number of scholars have dealt with the topic of human nature, and most of this literature focuses on narrow aspects rather than a more synoptic review and recasting of religious views.

Periods of attention to genetic developments within the religious community have tended to be followed by years of seeming inattention. Involvement has rarely been sustained. After an initial burst of writing in the 1960s, there was a decade during which very few theologians, ethicists, or religious communities dealt with genetics or genetic engineering. Then in the second half of the 1980s and early 1990s most of the ecumenical and denominational statements were produced. After another hiatus, there is again a wave of activity in the late 1990s both in scholarly works and a cluster of "second-generation" denominational resources. These latter works finally provide a far more thoughtful and in-depth treatment.

Religious attention to cloning and genetic patenting has not been sustained either. News of Dolly's creation and the speculation about the applicability of nuclear transfer technology to humans quickly galvanized many official bodies and religious ethicists into taking a position on human cloning. But after the initial few months of commentary during the first half of 1997 and the publication of a collection of essays in November of that year,[42] little else was written or published on the topic until a second collection of essays was issued in 2001. To my knowledge, very few bodies or persons offering a religious perspective commented on discussions and subsequent developments related to cloning or draft legislation to regulate cloning. Similarly, aside from the recommendations of a group of religious ethicists commissioned by Geron Corporation,[43] there has been little in the way of in-depth commentary from mainline religious thinkers or bodies about the religious implications of stem cell research. At the time I am writing, the groups within the religious community most inclined to express a point of view have done so because they believe that embryonic stem cells are inappropriate subjects of research, but this critique does not address issues related to stem cell applications.

In much the same way, there was a flurry of activity on genetic patenting in the early 1980s when the Supreme Court issued its precedent-breaking decision to allow the patenting of genetically altered organisms. Then in 1987, the antibiotechnology activist Jeremy Rifkin solicited signatures from religious leaders on a petition opposing the patenting of genetically altered animals. In 1995, the "Joint Appeal Against Human and Animal Patenting" was issued, but there was virtual silence on the topic in between these events. Despite these expressions of concern, those opposing patenting of life forms on religious grounds have been very slow to articulate adequately the theological and ethical grounding of their doing so. That there is at least a small body of literature expressing religious perspectives is more a result of the reactions the Joint Appeal generated within and outside the religious community than a commitment to develop a theological understanding of patenting. And it should also be noted that two of the three dialogues with religious thinkers on this topic were organized by secular organizations with theologically trained ethicists on staff, namely the American Association for the Advancement of Science and The Hastings Center.

Only a handful of religious thinkers, mostly Protestants from mainline denominations, regularly deal with issues related to genetic science. Many of the same people play multiple roles serving on denominational and ecumenical task forces, drafting resources for churches, and writing their own articles and books. As knowledgeable as this fraternity is—and virtually all of them are Caucasian and male—they represent a relatively narrow range of religious and ethical perspectives. Surprisingly and disappointingly, very few Catholic moral theologians have written extensively on genetics. And even fewer thinkers from non-Christian backgrounds have joined the discussions.

The relative absence of Jewish, Muslim, Hindu, or Buddhist voices and perspectives reflects a variety of factors. Not all faith traditions have developed methodologies and approaches for addressing contemporary bioethical and genetics issues. In some, there is even fundamental disagreement within the community as to whether sacred scripture should or can be used as the basis for claims about that community's view on topics in medical ethics, let alone biotechnology. The absence of a centralized ecclesiastical structure or an official body to speak for or commission a study or the development of positions has obviously been an impediment for many communities. Some—the Jewish normative tradition, for example—have placed great emphasis on discussion, dialogue, and interaction as the means to interpret texts to fit new circumstances,[44] and there have not been opportunities for this to occur. It is also understandable that thinkers situated in regions of the world distant from the centers of genetic research and genetic testing would be less concerned about these issues.

Ethical Discourse: Ethical and Prophetic Modes

In his book *Intersections: Science, Theology, and Ethics*, James Gustafson distinguishes among four complementary modes of ethics: ethical discourse, prophetic discourse, narrative discourse, and policy discourse.[45]

The first of these, ethical discourse, sets forth how one ought to act in particular circumstances, and more specifically, it evaluates the moral justification for particular courses of action. Prophetic and narrative discourses present broader questions about worldview, vision, and basic values. The former is more general than ethical discourse and generally takes two forms, indictments and utopian thinking, both of which tend to be framed in passionate, metaphorical language. Narrative ethics deals with the selection of stories and narratives appropriate for shaping moral ethos and character. Policy discourse involves more practical issues regarding alternative possibilities for public policy. Gustafson also emphasizes that none of the modes of discourse is sufficient: At different moments or for specific purposes one or another may be more appropriate.

Much of the religious literature on genetics does not easily fit into any of Gustafson's categories. It most closely approximates the model characterized as ethical discourse, but it tends to be broadly interpretive and descriptive rather than prescriptive. It is likely that the authors were motivated by the intent to establish normative boundaries for the applications of genetic science. Most of the literature, however, focuses primarily on identifying the meaning of genetic discoveries rather than on providing guidance on how to proceed. To put it another way, much of this body of works attempts to sensitize readers to the many issues that specific genetic research and applications raise rather than to recommend guidelines on how to resolve these dilemmas. Frequently, the authors "punt," underscoring the need for caution or for further societal discussion before proceeding, as for example in the writings on human germ-line interventions that will be heritable. While societal education and discourse are worthwhile goals in dealing with new technologies, it is extraordinarily difficult to find an appropriate forum and have a meaningful review. Moreover, why should the public or policymakers be expected to have greater wisdom than the professional ethicists unable or unwilling to offer guidance?

Another problem is that the level of abstraction at which norms are presented makes them difficult to apply as action guides. The ethical framework in the United Church of Canada's brief on genetics is typical of the level of generality and abstraction in these works. Among the principles it proposes are: life is a gift of ultimate value and must be so respected; human beings are essentially relational rather than individual; justice and compassion are at the heart of being human; and medical technologies must be carefully scrutinized for their costs to human beings and their utilization of scarce resources.[46] Other sets of guidelines are similarly abstract. Roger Shinn's six guidelines for evaluating genetic developments include the following: "Genetic investigation and practice directed toward healing are beneficent—provided they guard against excessive risk, rash denials of human frailty, and partisan definitions of normality";[47] "We can intervene [in nature], with due caution, to protec[t] significant values";[48] "An ethically responsible program of genetic research and practice . . . will recognize the mystery of selfhood and will seek to protect freedom-in-community";[49] and "Diversity is an asset to be treasured."[50] While norms so formulated can sensitize the religious community and decision makers as to values to take into account, they require far more intellectual development before they can be utilized to evaluate specific courses of action. Shinn quite appropriately characterizes his six guidelines as referring "less to precise decisions than to the personal and cultural climate in which decisions are made."[51] If this description were to be slightly rephrased so that the norms referred less to precise guidelines than to personal, ethical, and religious considerations for people of faith making decisions, it would be relevant to much of the literature contributed by religious thinkers.

Unfortunately, these general and abstract guidelines and principles are neither developed further nor applied to analyze specific issues. If religious ethics had proceeded to do so, it could have made a real contribution to dealing with the dilemmas that genetic applications raise. Virtually no religious ethicists have attempted to formulate middle axioms, let alone to evaluate specific issues in light of their principles and middle axioms. Middle axioms have been described as "more concrete than a universal ethical principle and less specific than a program that includes legislation and political strategy. They are the next steps that our own generation must take in fulfilling the purposes of God."[52] The failure to develop middle axioms has hampered efforts to "operationalize" religious concerns. Therefore none of the principles and norms identified in this literature can offer clear directions, priorities, or limitations for the application of genetic power. Instead, ethicists frequently affirm the need to take ethical considerations into account and to draw specific boundaries, but fail to offer models on how to do so. And when they reach conclusions, they often do so on the basis of moral intuition rather than moral reasoning.

Prophetic discourse is a second of Gustafson's categories. Characteristically prophetic ethics tend to be "macro" in orientation and to be occupied with the roots of what is perceived to be fundamentally and systematically wrong. This discourse usually is passionate and sometimes apocalyptic. It combines the marshalling of evidence to underscore an indictment with the use of metaphors and analogies to stir the hearers' emotions.[53] Some of the religious literature clearly aspires to engage in prophetic inquiry, but these works rarely do so successfully. In part, this reflects the difficulties of engaging in prophetic discourse in relationship to science and technology. In comparison with other subject matter, there is a greater need to base prophetic calls on clear analysis and arguments, in this case based on knowledge of scientific developments. This is not a simple task and only a few thinkers, the scientist and ethicist Leon Kass for one, have managed to do so.

In its 1991 resolution, "On Implications of Genetic Research and the Church's Response," the Presbyterian Church commits itself to engage in prophetic inquiry concerning the theological and ethical issues raised by the Human Genome Project. It defines prophetic inquiry as "the means by which we use the wisdom of modern technology and science integrated with the teachings of biblical tradition in order to move more fully toward God's kingdom of wholeness and justice."[54] However, the analyses of the potential challenges of genetic research, testing, and applications in this and many other of the resources does not differ noticeably from many secular evaluations. And particularly the resources developed by or for specific communities often are quite superficial and therefore lack the grounding on which to make a prophetic call.

Much of the public policy work on genetic developments has emanated from social policy or church and society units within the major denominations, some of whom are quite critical of some aspects of genetic development. A clear instance is the 1995 "Joint Appeal Against Human and Animal Patenting." One analyst, who is a former staff member of the United Methodist Board of Church and Society, defends this statement on the grounds that its proponents were using a prophetic argumentative framework. In his article, John Evans appears to assume that a prophetic orientation does not need to undergird or support its indictment by a clearly formulated argument, let alone reasoning based on knowledge of the subject matter.[55] While it is true that prophetic discourse differs in its mode of reasoning from more conventional ethical reasoning, I don't believe that this excuses sloppy thinking. Moreover, the very fact that society tends to be resistant to prophetic approaches would suggest the advisability of having accurate facts, careful ethical reasoning, and precise conclusions, particularly when dealing with a technical issue, such as genetic patenting. Otherwise, religious advocates are more likely to appear unknowing than prophetic.

One of the reasons that the religious response to genetics is less prophetic or even incisive than it might be is the failure to deal consistently and thoroughly with justice dimensions of the issues. The recognition that genetic discoveries and applications have significant justice implications does not translate into the development of a consistent justice trajectory in these works. And when justice concerns are brought to the fore, they are rarely addressed within an explicitly religious or theological context. Titles can be deceptive. For example, few of the essays in the collection *Genetics: Issues of Social Justice*[56] actually focus on justice issues. Moreover, like other norms and principles, the commitment to justice is often stated abstractly without clearly spelling out what it means or requires in a particular circumstance.

In addition, the treatment of justice issues rarely deals with the very important role that commercial interests play in shaping the priorities for genetic research and development and the implications of commercialization for the future of genetics. Various authors comment in passing that corporate aims and distributive justice might be incompatible,[57] but they have not spelled out or focused on this very important point. Even the religious critics of patenting focus primarily on the symbolic issues related to the patenting of life and its potential impact on human dignity. Their concerns with patenting regimes rarely address the larger issues of the influence of the marketplace over genetic developments. One of the most perceptive treatments of this topic occurs in a recent article in which Lisa Sowle Cahill evaluates the proposals of a group of ethicists advising a biotechnology company on human stem cell research. Cahill quite rightly points out that statements advocating "global distributive justice and equitable access," as does the work of the Geron Ethics Advisory Board, will not have much meaning unless the ethicists deal with what she terms "the new biotech world order." This is because social justice commitments to equitable access to genetic services, especially for those whose needs are greatest, face new and daunting challenges in a global market economy."[58] In her commentary, she notes that the biotechnology corporations driving genetic development are likely to derive greater profits in a global context of vastly unequal access to health care and other human goods. I agree with her analysis and believe that this topic requires priority attention from religious ethicists addressing genetics.

Public Theology and Policy Discourse

Ronald Thiemann has defined public theology as "faith seeking to understand the relation between Christian convictions and the broader social and cultural context within which the Christian community lives."[59] Others, such as Max Stackhouse, have emphasized that public theology seeks to give ethical guidance to the structures and policies of public life.[60] Both of these are relevant to the various ecumenical and denominational initiatives on genetics that have taken place during the past twenty years. Much of the literature addressing ethical issues arising from the genetics revolution does not clearly specify the intended audience and appears at least implicitly to address the broader society. Several publications explicitly try to reach beyond their own members to inform a broader public, including policymakers.

Much of the thrust of this public theology is more to underscore the need for public discussions and societal decision making than to prescribe particular policy directions. Positions of religious thinkers and agencies on two of the most controversial issues, human germ-line engineering and somatic cell nuclear cloning, for example, typically emphasize the need for a moratorium so as to permit ethical reflection necessary for developing guidelines. Although the various religious congregations and educational institutions in this country potentially constitute one of the largest forums for ethical deliberation, the role proposed for the church or religious communions is surprisingly modest. While much of this literature eloquently justifies the religious community addressing the genetic revolution, it usually does not envisage any religious body taking a leadership role in developing national policy on this topic. Instead the various statements and works confine the role of churches to monitoring and participating in governmental, legislative, and public policy debates.

There have also been several instances when religious bodies sought to influence the formation of public policy. One example of the latter was the 1980 letter to President Carter calling for the establishment of adequate mechanisms for public review and oversight of genetic engineering. This letter then led to the broadening of the mandate of the President's Commission for the Study of Ethical Problems in Medicine and Biomedical and Behavioral Research to genetic engineering and invitations to religious thinkers to participate in its deliberations. The 1995 "Joint Appeal Against Human and Animal Patenting" constitutes another initiative, perhaps more to record the religious communities' discomfort with the direction of patent policies than the expectation of changing them. In 1997, several religious bodies, as well as religious scholars, issued statements intended to influence the shaping of public policy on human cloning through the statements, resolutions, and testimony before the National Bioethics Advisory Commission.

The interface between faith, Christian and non-Christian, and public theology on genetics reflects the recognition of the significance of the genetics revolution for contemporary and future generations and the unprecedented nature of the choices it brings. As early as 1984, a publication of the National Council of Churches in the U.S.A. expressed the conviction that discoveries in human genetics may revolutionize our fundamental understandings of the world and the role of humanity. This publication anticipates that this turning point may have implications as far-reaching as Copernicus's finding that the earth revolved around the sun, Darwin's theory of evolution, and Einstein's theory of matter.[61] The capacity to genetically engineer forms of life and reshape human nature may eventually propel us toward the role of co-creators, hopefully with the recognition of our finitude and creatureliness. Given their analysis of the broad societal implications of genetic developments, the religious community gravitates toward the public arena both to raise various issues and to seek resolution of them. In taking these initiatives, religious communities and thinkers hold the conviction that "The church [religious community] has significant and distinctive things to say about a society wrestling with the questions and the meaning of genetic developments,"[62] and they are usually correct about this. The activist character of American religion also propels faith bodies into social and political life as a manifestation of their sense of their religious call or witness in society. In an earlier work, I observed the following about Christian faith and politics: "A faith that is social, ethical, and incarnational . . . cannot countenance the liberal delineation of politics and religion as unrelated to each other. Such a separation of faith and politics, moreover, contradicts the biblical perspective that time and again affirms God as the ultimate source of meaning, authority, and inspiration over all spheres of life."[63]

A decade or so ago several books and articles anticipated the development of a "naked public square" stripped of religious perspectives,[64] but this does not appear to be the case with regard to religious input on various issues related to the genetics revolution. Religious participation in discussions about genetics has generally been welcomed and sometimes even solicited. This reflects, at least at some junctures, the growing sense in the public that developments like human cloning have authentic religious dimensions. Of course, there have been critical voices, some from the scientific community, arguing that "ancient theological scruples" have no appropriate role in the formation of public policy on genetic issues. The National Bioethics Advisory Commission's (NBAC) justification of why it invited religious thinkers to offer their views on human cloning provides a powerful rejoinder to these claims. NBAC acknowledged that the U.S. Constitution prohibits the establishment of policies that are solely motivated by religious belief, but explained that NBAC felt that religious perspectives were especially important "because religious traditions shape the moral views of many U.S. citizens and religious teachings over the centuries have provided an important source of ideas and inspiration."[65] NBAC goes on to state that "Although in a pluralistic society particular religious views cannot be determinative for public policy decisions that bind everyone, policy makers should understand and show respect for diverse moral ideas regarding the acceptability of cloning human beings."[66] Not only did NBAC set aside time to hear a diverse group of religious ethicists, it also devoted a chapter of its report to analyzing their viewpoints and recommendations.

While affirming the public witness role of the religious community, I have been critical about the way in which it is sometimes executed. Elsewhere I have suggested several guidelines for public theology growing out of my critique of the Joint Appeal. First, for public theology to be consistent with the nature and mission of a religious actor, I believe it should proceed from a clear religious rationale and reflect the priorities of the communions it is representing. In order to speak for, rather than to, the religious community, public theology should represent the views of a wide cross-section of members of a faith communion and not just its leadership. To do so, it requires systematic education and wide-ranging consultation with members in advance of any public initiatives. Second, to be appropriate, public theology should be timely and at the very least explain why the religious community or communion has decided to address a specific issue in the public arena. Third, it is important that public theology be well reasoned, informed, and understandable to persons within both the religious and secular communities. When public theology appeals to theological beliefs, even when the beliefs are not widely shared, the logical relationship between the beliefs and the conclusions should be comprehensible to believer and nonbeliever alike.[67] Fourth, to be credible, public theology should exhibit knowledge of relevant research and data related to the subject it is addressing. This is particularly the case on topics related to science and technology. Fifth, if public theology aims at changing public policy, it needs to be clear about what it is advocating as well as what it is criticizing.

To what extent did the public policy initiatives of religious spokespersons on genetic patenting and human cloning discussed in this essay conform to these criteria? My analysis of the Joint Appeal illustrates that it did not meet any of these conditions. Opponents of patenting did claim a religious grounding, but it was poorly articulated. Moreover, the Joint Appeal did not build on a long-term and consistent concern with patenting issues in the religious community. Science and technology, let alone genetic issues or patenting, are barely on the agenda of most religious leaders and communions. Far from there being a religious consensus over patenting, those most knowledgeable about the topic tended to disagree with the position and theological rationale of the Joint Appeal and/or argued that the patenting of life forms is peripheral to the primary issues before the religious community. The Joint Appeal was also problematic because it certainly was not timely or related to specific developments in patent policy. Further, with a very small number of exceptions, the religious participants in the genetic patenting debate were not well informed about the specifics of patent law or the status of genetic patenting, and this undercut their credibility. Nor did the critique of the Joint Appeal make clear the specific changes the coalition was advocating.

The religious witness on cloning came somewhat closer, particularly in being timely. The statements issued by various religious bodies, as well as the articles and testimony of religious ethicists, expressed a clear religious rationale that was understandable both to their own members and to the wider public. While it is difficult to know whether any of the thinkers or agencies represented the views of a strong cross-section of members of their communion, some did seek broader membership support after the fact. In contrast with the Joint Appeal, whose timing represents something of a mystery, the input on cloning came at a point of public attention and discussion after the announcement of the cloning of a lamb, but then dropped away as Congress actually considered the text of specific bills. The statements addressing cloning were far more well reasoned, informed, and understandable to persons within the religious and secular communities than the Joint Appeal text. In addition, the cloning critics who argued for either a prohibition or a moratorium generally were clear about what they were advocating.

Engaging in public theology so as to offer ethical guidance to the structures and policies of public life requires making religious discourse publicly accessible. To be clear about the religious basis of the claims made and the policies advocated while communicating with a broader public offers quite a challenge. Utilizing the experience of religious thinkers in the field of bioethics, several secular ethicists have expressed concerns about the feasibility of translating religious discourse into a common moral language appropriate to an interdisciplinary and public audience. Leon Kass notes that there is little choice but for religious ethicists to leave their special insights at the door and to adopt secular categories and terminologies.[68] Another problem, according to the philosopher Jeffrey Stout, is that there is no universal and neutral ethical language, no "Esperanto" into which theological formulations can be translated. Stout is not unduly disturbed because he does not infer that talk of God is irrelevant to the public life or to the society's ethical discourse.[69]

In contrast with some of the secular ethicists, Lisa Sowle Cahill argued that there is not an independent realm of secular or philosophical discourse that is privileged because it is more reasonable, neutral, or objective, and less tradition-bound than religious discourse. Instead she pointed out that all ethicists attempt to speak out of but beyond a particular tradition. According to Cahill, it is best to construe public discourse "as embodying a commitment to civil exchanges among traditions, many of which have an overlapping membership, and which meet on the basis of common concerns."[70] She recommended that religiously motivated spokespersons develop policy initiatives on the basis of moral quandaries, moral sensibilities, moral images, and moral vocabulary shared among a variety of religious and moral traditions. If they did so, she anticipated that theologians and religious groups could contribute to public discourse by serving a critical function and cutting through cultural assumptions.[71]

Public theology related to genetic issues has generally focused on moral dilemmas, values, sensitivities, and images, utilizing both faith specific language and a shared moral vocabulary. Faith language on genetics and biotechnology has usually been comprehensible precisely because it has transcended a particular community's positions and beliefs. By doing so, it has offered perspectives congenial to supporters of other moral traditions, including some forms of secular humanism. Rather than "God talk," religious ethicists have tended to ground their concerns and objections in terminology and concepts consistent with human rights principles and the ideals of a democratic society. They have emphasized such norms such as protecting human dignity, assuring nondiscrimination, and promoting substantive justice and fairness, while reasoning out of but also beyond specific religious traditions.

Has this approach imposed a cost? Or to ask this question in another way: Have theologians and ethicists consciously sacrificed God talk so as to be more comprehensible to a wider public? My answer is not very often. In part, this derives from an increasingly higher threshold of acceptance of theological language in the public arena on some of these issues, cloning for example, than was anticipated in the earlier discussions about the public role of religion arising out of bioethics. The acknowledgment that many genetic discoveries raise religious questions has helped legitimate an explicitly religious presence in public discourse. The diffuse sense of anxiety about the implications of genetic engineering, especially applications directly affecting persons, may also contribute to openness to religious actors because they are viewed as representatives of a moral authority.

There is yet another reason why contributing to public discussions has not entailed stripping away theological layers of discourse. Most religious thinkers, even when writing for a religious audience, have placed their analysis of genetic discoveries primarily within an ethical rather than a theological framework. As noted, theological interpretations of the implications of genetics have lagged behind concerns with ethical dilemmas. This reflects a variety of factors, among them the difficulties and complexities of understanding genetic developments through traditional theological approaches and methodologies.

Distinctiveness of Religious Ethics

Are there specific approaches, sensitivities, or criteria that distinguish religious and secular ethicists? While religious communities and thinkers certainly did not speak with one voice on these issues, I believe that there were important shared themes and affinities, even when these works refrained from using "God language." To list some of these, religious thinkers often raise broader and more significant issues than many of the secular commentators. Despite their many differences in specifics and the rationale for arguing them, the various religious thinkers whose views were discussed in this study shared a strong commitment to moral and theological analysis of technological development so as to bring science under the guidance of ethical choice. In a society where risk-benefit analysis tends to be the currency of public policy analysis, the religious community offers an alternative vision based on principles of human dignity and worth. Moreover, in contrast with those who claim that decisions about genetic developments should be left solely to the individual, moral theologians consistently argue that societal well-being goes beyond questions of private ethics to wider issues of public decision making and morality. Religious thinkers are also more likely to have sensitivities for the justice implications of genetics, gene patenting, and cloning, particularly for those persons and groups who are unable or unlikely to speak for themselves.

That religious thinkers frequently raise "big-picture" issues is both a strength and weakness of their work. One of the contributions religious perspectives provide is to offer broad frameworks of understanding and commitment so necessary to deal with these complex issues. A religious centering by its very nature offers a vision in which persons are responsible beyond their own self-interest to the ultimate source of grounding of their lives and being. Resources written by the religious community typically emphasize a need for science and technology to serve the welfare, common good, and fulfillment of the broader human society. A member of the National Bioethics Advisory Commission acknowledged his appreciation for the testimony and perspectives of the religious community on cloning for just this reason.[72] The symbols and metaphors that religious thinkers use that complicate their ethical analysis may also incline them to deal with the broader implications of specific discoveries and applications.

That religious ethicists tend to go beyond an individualistic perspective may reflect their own sense of connectedness to a community, a tradition, and ultimately to the divine. Religious thinkers also often have a social conception of personhood. In contrast with the secular approach based on individual rights and on notions of reproductive and medical privacy, many religious thinkers hold up the importance of a framework that places individuals within the context of the community and upholds the importance of considerations of the common good. In a commentary on the ethical and theological considerations related to cloning written for the United Church of Christ, Karen Lebacqz wrote the following about the Christian vision:

In that vision, all individual rights are always concordant with a fundamental commitment to the good, including the demands of justice. No one has "rights" independent of a concern for the social whole and for the well-being of God's creation. All "rights" involve responsibilities. While it is difficult to delineate exactly the range of these responsibilities, or the limits that they might place on the exercise of individual rights, we know that unless we take a relational view of the world, we fail to capture the purposes of a God who so loved us that God sent God's only begotten so that all people might have life and have it abundantly.[73]

Lisa Sowle Cahill made an eloquent appeal in her testimony to the National Bioethics Advisory Commission to go beyond the confines of the principles of autonomy, individuality, and individual freedom to consider other social goods, particularly the interdependence of all in the society we create for ourselves and our children. Like many other religious thinkers, Cahill's frame of reference was the character of a good society and what we can do concretely to move in the appropriate direction.[74] Likewise, Abdulaziz Sachedina stated in his testimony that the central ethical question for Islam was how cloning might affect interhuman or interpersonal relationships. He asked whether human advancement in biotechnology-created relationships would jeopardize the very foundation of human community.[75]

While I am sometimes critical of the failure of religious thinkers to focus more systematically and in greater depth on justice issues, for example in the discussion of genetic patenting, I would like to acknowledge that religious thinkers generally are more sensitive than their secular counterparts to justice considerations. Justice traditions within the religious community and concern with the needs of those lacking a voice in decision making play a role in the response to genetic technologies and cloning. Also, the understanding of justice and its requirements is significantly broader among religious ethicists. Many secular philosophers and ethicists, particularly those influenced by the "Georgetown mantra" based on the *Principles of Biomedical Ethics*,[76] identify justice as only one of several principles central to biomedical ethics. They often treat justice as of less importance than other principles, particularly respect for the autonomy of patients. Justice is also typically explicated in the secular literature primarily in terms of fairness in one-on-one relationships, as between a provider and patient. In contrast, religious ethicists view justice as constitutive of systems as well as individual relationships. They are more likely to question the basis on which broader societal patterns of benefits and burdens are distributed. The work of religious thinkers often goes beyond principles of formal justice and empirical research dealing with various risks, costs, and benefits to a more egalitarian approach to justice. When religious ethicists deal with justice issues, they tend to emphasize either the need for equitable distribution of the goods of life or preferential access for those who are disadvantaged. The 1992 United Methodist resolution, for example, mentions the importance of genetic therapies being available to all members of society, and not just the wealthy.[77] Nevertheless, much of the discussion of justice issues is quite brief and cursory in the religious literature on genetics. Understandings of the requirements of justice often remain more implicit than explicit, and concerns are rarely developed adequately.

Justice themes were more prominent in some of the religious commentary on cloning. Again, to quote Lebacqz, "Justice requires that we see ourselves as bound in a covenant of life with life, in which individual freedom and choice . . . [are] always coupled with a sense of social responsibility and a particular concern for the poor and oppressed. This is what it means to have a biblical perspective on justice."[78] Lebacqz also emphasizes that a Christian perspective evaluates technological achievements in the context of global justice. Because cloning will not be available to the poor and oppressed around the globe, but only to the wealthy and privileged, she concludes that it violates the demands of a wide-ranging biblical justice.[79] The United Church of Christ's statement/resolution on cloning specifically mentions the denomination's commitment to justice and views cloning through this lens: "When the world groans with hunger, when children are stunted from chronic malnutrition, when people die of famine by the thousands every day— when this is the reality of the world in which we live, the development of any more technologies to suit the desires of those who are relatively privileged, secure, and comfortable seems to fly in the face of fundamental claims of justice."[80] Likewise, Elliott Dorff and several other religious commentators were concerned about the implications of cloning on socioeconomic divisions within our society.[81] In her testimony to the National Bioethics Advisory Commission, Nancy Duff urged that if we proceed with research into human cloning that we be mindful of those who are most likely to be exploited and specifically mentioned the importance of protecting women, racial and ethic minorities, prisoners, and the poor against exploitation.[82] The statement from the United Methodist Genetic Science Task Force has very similar language.[83]

In contrast with secular ethicists' tendency to emphasize the positive potential contributions of genetic technologies, many religious thinkers evince what might be described as a presumption of caution. By this I mean that they place greater priority on anticipating and preventing potential problems than on favoring technologies and applications because they may bring future benefits. Writing for the Evangelical Lutheran Church in America, Roger Willer characterized this approach as "critical engagement" and explained that it means that Christians generally support genetic science but are required to evaluate any particular genetic discovery or application according to criteria informed by faith and Christian sources.[84] This difference in emphasis is considerable when comparing the religious approach with the comments of some secular thinkers on cloning. Some secular thinkers, for example, argued that it would be premature to close off research opportunities on the grounds that only a few people are likely to reap benefits and claimed that it would be prejudicial to ban an entire line of research because of possible unethical applications. In contrast, religious thinkers tended to be more mindful of those who were likely to be harmed than those who were likely to benefit and to seek to protect important societal values, even if this requires constraints on science and technology.

Yet this presumption of caution has its limits because of the generally hopeful and supportive approach to genetics. The dilemmas intrinsic to balancing hopes and fears—accepting the benefits while still offering a warning about some of the likely consequences—are reflected in the writings of Philip Hefner. In one of his essays on genetics, Hefner offers a perceptive critique of the prevailing worldview in our society, including how it impinges on genetics, and suggests that the Christian faith and theological perspectives can offer a constructive alternative.[85] Hefner characterizes the tapestry of ideas, commitments, values, hopes, and fears that currently forms the background of what we say and do as a "fix-it" or "repair-it" mentality. He argues that this approach to life reflects our innately co-creating and nature-shaping human nature, but it also results in a failure to acknowledge our status as creatures in nature with fundamental limitations and flaws. Another problem with the "fix-it" disposition, according to Hefner, is its tendency to segregate and ostracize those who deviate from the norm and to treat persons with disabilities as needing to be fixed rather than valuable in their own right. Hefner finds corrections in Christian theological perspectives on finitude, ambiguity, and failure, and most importantly, in the belief that humans are weak and sinful.

But does the religious literature on genetics, specifically those works written by Christians, offer a real alternative to the prevailing "fix-it" or "hammer-and-nails" approach to life? My answer would have to be not really. Yes, there are some very significant cautions about proceeding with remaking human nature or the world around us. Hefner, for example, warns that the Human Genome Project as well as the growing emphasis on genetic testing reflect the prevailing worldview. But the theological conceptions of humanity as co-creators or partners in completing or correcting the flaws in the creation, ironically popularized through some of Hefner's own writing, tend to support, even sacralize, efforts at genetic engineering. Theologians and ethicists who refrain from using these images are little different in their underlying views on genetics. Moreover, most of the religious analysis of genetics shares the societal desire for health and physical well-being that Hefner attributes to the prevailing worldview, as well as the strong hope that genetics will significantly contribute to healing and improved health. Thus, despite their discomfort with the impact of genetic technologies, few, if any, religious ethicists stand apart from this consensus and oppose these developments. Human cloning constitutes the one exception where the religious community almost unanimously uttered the "prophetic no."

Conclusion

During the past twenty years a variety of religious bodies and thinkers have recognized and responded to the genetics revolution. Their work has made an important contribution to societal efforts to identify and begin to grapple with the choices and dilemmas arising from genetic discoveries and applications. It is quite wide ranging in the topics and concerns it addresses. Most are Christian in background, but there are also signs of increasing interest among Jewish and a few Muslim ethicists. The major contribution of this literature has been to sensitize and stimulate the moral imagination of the religious and secular publics and to expand their ethical horizons. They have shown that genetics is relevant to the realms of ethics and theology as well as science and medicine. By identifying the values and commitments that genetic discoveries challenge, this literature makes clear that nothing less is at stake than the moral compass and fundamental humanity of our own society and that of future societies.

Twenty-five years ago, James Gustafson observed that theology rarely yields precise and concrete directives for bioethical decision making.[86] On a similar note, in 1990 Lisa Sowle Cahill noted that even within the religious community, theology is more likely to affirm fundamental values and commitments relevant to the bioethical decision making of religious persons than to yield specific norms.[87] The same could be said of the ethical literature on genetics and biotechnology subsequently written by religious thinkers. Few of the works offer specific guidance toward resolving the many ethical dilemmas and unprecedented choices resulting from genetic developments. Nor do they provide norms, methodologies, or guidelines to use in making these determinations. The various thinkers do not illuminate where to draw the precise boundary between genetic interventions representing responsible expressions of human stewardship, co-creation, or partnership with the divine and those that are extensions of human hubris or pride. Instead, it can be said that the greatest value of these works is more in the issues they raise than the answers they provide.

Is this role sufficient? I think not. I have greater aspirations for religious thinkers dealing with biotechnology. Given the magnitude of the issues—as set forth in the various analyses of the unprecedented challenges and choices related to genetic developments in these works— it is not enough to stimulate the moral imagination. Unless religious ethicists can offer guidance on how to respond to these developments or, at the least, offer a normative approach, they may be bypassed by their members and the broader society alike.

NOTES

1. This chapter is based on Audrey R. Chapman, *Unprecedented Choices: Religious Ethics at the Frontiers of Genetic Science*, copyright © 1999 Augsburg Fortress (ISBN 0-8006-3181-1). Reprinted by permission.

2. Letter from Dr. Claire Randall, General Secretary, National Council of Churches, Rabbi Bernard Mandelbaum, General Secretary, Synagogue Council of America, and Bishop Thomas Kelly, General Secretary, United States Catholic Conference to President Carter, 20 June 1980. The letter is reproduced in President's Commission for the Study of Ethical Problems in Medicine and Biomedical and Behavioral Research, *Splicing Life: The Social and Ethical Issues of Genetic Engineering with Human Beings* (Washington, D.C.: U.S. Government Printing Office, 1982), Appendix B, p. 95.

3. Letter from three general secretaries, *Splicing Life*, p. 96.

4. Letter from three general secretaries, *Splicing Life*, p. 96.

5. Audrey R. Chapman, *Unprecedented Choices: Religious Ethics at the Frontiers of Genetic Science* (Minneapolis, Minn.: Fortress Press, 1999).

6. Robert Russell, executive director of the Center for Theology and the Natural Sciences, was so quoted in "To Clone or Not to Clone," *Christian Century* 114, no. 10 (19–26 March 1997): 286–88, at 286.

7. This chronology of ecumenical discussions on genetics follows Roger L. Shinn, "Genetics, Ethics, and Theology: Ecumenical Discussions," in *Genetics: Issues of Social Justice*, ed. Ted Peters (Cleveland, Ohio: The Pilgrim Press, 1998), pp. 122–43.

8. World Council of Churches, Church and Society, *Manipulating Life: Ethical Issues in Genetic Engineering* (Geneva: Church and Society, World Council of Churches, 1982).

9. World Council of Churches, Church and Society, *Biotechnology: Its Challenges to the Church and the World* (Geneva: Church and Society, World Council of Churches, 1989).

10. National Council of the Churches of Christ in the U.S.A., *Human Life and the New Genetics: A Report of a Task Force Commissioned by the National Council of Churches of Christ in the U.S.A.* (New York: National Council of Churches, 1980).

11. Panel of Bioethical Concerns, *Genetic Engineering: Social and Ethical Consequences*, ed. Frank M. Harron (New York: Pilgrim Press, 1984).

12. National Council of the Churches of Christ in the U.S.A., "Genetic Science for Human Benefit: A Policy Statement of the National Council of the Churches of Christ in the U.S.A." Approved by the Governing Council, 1986.

13. Congregation for the Doctrine of the Faith, *Instruction on Respect for Human Life in its Origin and on the Dignity of Procreation* (*Donum Vitae*), 1987. The text is reproduced in Kevin D. O'Rourke, O.P., J.C.D., S.T.M. and Philip Boyle, *Medical Ethics: Sources of Catholic Teaching*, 2d ed. (Washington, D.C.: Georgetown University Press, 1993).

14. John Paul II, "The Ethics of Genetic Manipulation," *Origins* 13 (1983): 386–89.

15. Catholic Health Association of the United States, *Human Genetics: Ethical Issues in Genetic Testing, Counseling, and Therapy* (St. Louis: The Catholic Health Association of the United States, 1990).

16. Working Party of the Catholic Bishops' Joint Committee on Bioethical Issues, *Genetic Intervention on Human Subjects* (London: Catholic Bishops' Joint Committee on Bioethical Issues, 1996).

17. Presbyterian Church (U.S.A.), "The Covenant of Life and the Caring Community and Covenant and Creation: Theological Reflections on Contraception and Abortion," Policy Statements and Recommendations Adopted by the 195th General Assembly, 1983 (Louisville, Ky.: The Office of the General Assembly, 1983).

18. "The Covenant of Life and the Caring Community," adopted by the 195th (1983) General Assembly, Presbyterian Church (U.S.A.), *Social Policy Compilation* (Louisville, Ky.: Advisory Committee on Social Witness Policy, 1992), pp. 97 and 846. The resolution of the 202d (1990) General Assembly, which is untitled in the compilation, is on p. 776.

19. "Genetic Engineering," Reports on Christian Action, *Minutes of the General Synod 1988* (New York: Reformed Church of America, 1988).

20. Pronouncement, "Church and Genetic Engineering," *Minutes, Seventeenth General Synod, United Church of Christ* (St. Louis: United Church Resources, 1991), pp. 45–47.

21. Resolution, "The Church and Reproductive Technologies," *Minutes, Seventeenth General Synod, United Church of Christ* (St. Louis: United Church Resources, 1991), pp. 45–47.

22. "New Developments in Genetic Science," *The Book of Resolutions of the United Methodist Church* (Nashville, Tenn.: The United Methodist Publishing House, 1992), pp. 325–38.

23. "A Brief to the Royal Commission on New Reproductive Technologies on Behalf of The United Church of Canada prepared by The Division of Mission in Canada," approved by the Executive of the Division of Mission, 17 January 1991.

24. John P. Burgess, ed., *In Whose Image? Faith, Science, and the New Genetics* (Louisville, Ky.: Geneva Press for the Office of Theology and Worship, Congregational Ministries Division, Presbyterian Church U.S.A., 1998), p. xi.

25. Cynthia B. Cohen, Chair, Committee on Medical Ethics, Episcopal Diocese of Washington, *Wrestling with the Future: Our Genes and Our Choices*, prepublication manuscript, 1998.

26. Roger A. Willer, ed., *Genetic Testing and Screening: Critical Engagement at the Intersection of Faith and Science* (Minneapolis, Minn.: Kirk House Publishers, Division for Church in Society, Evangelical Church in America, 1998).

27. Donald Bruce and Ann Bruce, *Engineering Genesis: The Ethics of Genetic Engineering in Non-Human Species* (London: Earthscan Publications for the Working Group of the Society, Religion and Technology Project, Church of Scotland, 1998).

28. Roger A. Willer, "Introduction," in *Genetic Testing and Screening*, ed. Willer, pp. 5–12, at p. 5.

29. John F. Kilner, Rebecca D. Pentz, and Frank E. Young, eds., *Genetic Ethics: Do the Ends Justify the Genes?* (Grand Rapids, Mich.: Wm. B. Eerdmans Publishing Co., 1997); Ted Peters, *Genetics: Issues of Social Justice* (Cleveland, Ohio: The Pilgrim Press, 1998).

30. Ronald Cole-Turner, *The New Genesis: Theology and the Genetic Revolution* (Louisville, Ky.: Westminster/John Knox Press, 1993), p. 109.

31. Ronald Cole-Turner and Brent Waters, *Pastoral Genetics: Theology and Care at the Beginning of Life* (Cleveland, Ohio: Pilgrim Press, 1996).

32. Barry Freundel, "Personal Religious Positions Individually Expressed: Judaism," in *On the New Frontiers of Genetics and Religion*, ed. J. Robert Nelson (Grand Rapids, Mich.: Wm. B. Eerdmans Publishing Company, 1994), 120–35.

33. Roger Lincoln Shinn, *The New Genetics: Challenges for Science, Faith, and Politics* (Wakefield, R.I. and London: Moyer Bell, 1996).

34. Shinn, *The New Genetics*, p. 89.

35. Ted Peters, *Playing God? Genetic Determinism and Human Freedom* (New York: Routledge, 1997).

36. Peters, *Playing God?* p. x.

37. Peters, *Playing God?* p. xvii.

38. Jan Christian Heller, *Human Genome Research and the Challenge of Contingent Future Persons* (Omaha, Nebr.: Creighton University Press, 1996).

39. Ronald Cole-Turner, ed., *Human Cloning: Religious Responses* (Louisville, Ky.: Westminster/John Knox Press, 1997); Ronald Cole-Turner, ed., *Religion and the Remaking of Humanity* (Harrisburg, Penn.: Trinity Press International, 2001).

40. ITEST Workshop, *Patenting of Biological Entities: Proceedings of the ITEST Workshop, October 1996* (St. Louis: ITEST Faith/Science Press, 1997).

41. Audrey R. Chapman, ed., *Perspectives on Genetic Patenting: Religion, Science, and Industry in Dialogue* (Washington, D.C.: American Association for the Advancement of Science, 1999).

42. Cole-Turner, *Human Cloning.*

43. Geron Ethics Advisory Board (Karen Lebacqz, chair, Michael M. Mendiola, Ted Peters, Ernlé W. D. Young, and Laurie Zoloth-Dorfman), "Research with Human Embryonic Stem Cells: Ethical Considerations," *Hasting Center Report* 29, no. 2 (1999): 31–36.

44. Noam J. Zohar, *Alternatives in Jewish Bioethics* (Albany: State University of New York Press, 1997), pp. 8–9.

45. James M. Gustafson, *Intersections: Science, Theology, and Ethics* (Cleveland, Ohio: The Pilgrim Press, 1996), pp. 35–55.

46. The Division of Mission in Canada, "A Brief to the Royal Commission on New Reproductive Technologies on behalf of The United Church of Canada," approved by the Executive of the Division of Mission, 17 January 1991, p. 3.

47. Roger Lincoln Shinn, *The New Genetics: Challenges for Science, Faith, and Politics* (Wakefield, R.I. and London: Moyer Bell, 1996), p. 108.

48. Shinn, *The New Genetics*, p. 110.

49. Shinn, *The New Genetics*, p. 112.

50. Shinn, *The New Genetics*, pp.114–15.

51. Shinn, *The New Genetics*, pp.120–21.

52. John C. Bennett, *Christian Ethics and Social Policy* (New York: Charles Scribner's Sons, 1946), pp. 76–77, as quoted in J. Philip Wogaman, *Christian Moral Judgment* (Louisville, Ky.: Westminster/John Knox Press, 1989), p. 49.

53. Gustafson, *Intersections*, p. 41.

54. Presbyterian Church (U.S.A.), 202d General Assembly (1990), "On the Implications of Genetic Research and the Church's Response," in *Social Policy Compilation* (Louisville, Ky.: Advisory Committee on Social Witness Policy, 1992), pp. 775–77.

55. John H. Evans, "The Uneven Playing Field of the Dialogue on Patenting," in *Perspectives on Gene Patenting: Religion, Science, and Industry in Dialogue,* ed. Audrey R. Chapman (Washington, D.C.: American Association for the Advancement of Science, 1999), pp. 57–74.

56. Ted Peters, *Genetics: Issues of Social Justice* (Cleveland, Ohio: The Pilgrim Press, 1998).

57. See, for example, the comments in Bruce and Bruce, *Engineering Genesis*, pp. 259–63.

58. Cahill, "The New Biotech World Order," pp. 45–46.

59. Ronald F. Thiemann, *Constructing a Public Theology: The Church in a Pluralistic Culture* (Louisville, Ky.: Westminster/John Knox Press, 1991), p. 21.

60. Max Stackhouse, *Public Theology and Political Economy* (Grand Rapids, Mich.: W. B. Eerdmans Pub. Co. for Commission on Stewardship, National Council of the Churches of Christ in the U.S.A., 1987), p. xi.

61. Panel on Bioethical Concerns, *Genetic Engineering: Social and Ethical Consequences*, ed. Frank M. Harron (New York: Pilgrim Press, 1984), p. 20.

62. Roger A. Willer, "Introduction," in *Genetic Testing and Screening: Critical Engagement at the Intersection of Faith and Science,* ed. Roger A. Willer (Minneapolis, Minn.: Kirk House Publishers for the Evangelical Lutheran Church in America), p. 7.

63. Audrey R. Chapman, *Faith, Power, and Politics: Political Ministry in Mainline Churches* (New York: The Pilgrim Press, 1991), p. 44.

64. Richard John Neuhaus, *The Naked Public Square: Religion and Democracy in America* (Grand Rapids, Mich.: William B. Eerdmans Publishing Company, 1984).

65. *Cloning Human Beings*, p. 7.

66. *Cloning Human Beings*, p. 7.

67. Ronald Cole-Turner, "The Theological Status of DNA: A Contribution to the Debate over Gene Patenting," revised version of a paper written for the AAAS Dialogue Group on Gene Patenting that was originally presented on 13 March 1997.

68. Leon R. Kass, "Practicing Ethics: Where's the Action?" *Hastings Center Report* 20 (January/February 1990): 5–11.

69. Jeffrey Stout, *Ethics After Babel: The Languages of Morals and Their Discontents* (Boston: Beacon Press, 1988), p. 187.

70. Lisa Sowle Cahill, "Can Theology Have a Role in 'Public' Bioethical Discourse?" *Hastings Center Report* 20, no. 4, special supplement (July/August 1990): S10–14, at S10.

71. Cahill, "Can Theology Have a Role?" pp. 10–14.

72. Conversation with Tom Murray, 24 September 1997.

73. Karen Lebacqz, "Some Ethical and Theological Considerations about Cloning," unpublished background paper written for the United Church of Christ Genetics Working Group, 1998, quoted with the permission of the author.

74. Lisa Sowle Cahill, "Testimony to the National Bioethics Advisory Commission," Washington, D.C., 14 March 1997, Eberlin Reporting Service, p. 50.

75. Aziz Sachedina, "Testimony to the National Bioethics Advisory Commission," Washington, D.C., 14 March 1997, Eberlin Reporting Service, pp. 16–21.

76. Tom L. Beauchamp and James F. Childress, *Principles of Biomedical Ethics*, 4th ed. (New York: Oxford University Press, 1994).

77. United Methodist Church, "New Developments in Genetic Science," *The Book of Resolutions of the United Methodist Church* (Nashville: The United Methodist Publishing House, 1992), pp. 325–38.

78. Lebacqz, "Some Ethical and Theological Considerations."

79. Lebacqz, "Some Ethical and Theological Considerations."

80. "Resolution on the Cloning of Mammalian Species to the 21st General Synod of the United Church of Christ," adopted July 1997. The text was made available to the author, who served as a member of the drafting committee.

81. Elliott Dorff, "Testimony to the National Bioethics Advisory Commission," Washington, D.C., 14 March 1997, Eberlin Reporting Service, p. 2.

82. Nancy Duff, "Testimony to the National Bioethics Advisory Commission, Washington, D.C., 13 March 1997, Eberlin Reporting Service, p. 6.

83. Statement from the United Methodist Genetic Science Task Force.

84. Roger A. Willer, "Introduction," in *Genetic Testing and Screening*, p. 8.

85. Philip Hefner, "The Genetic 'Fix': Challenges to Christian Faith and Community," in *Genetic Testing and Screening*, ed. Roger A. Willer, pp. 73–93.

86. James M. Gustafson, *The Contributions of Theology to Medical Ethics* (Milwaukee, Wisc.: Marquette University Theology Department, 1975), cited in Cahill, "Can Theology Have a Role in 'Public' Bioethical Discourse?" p. S11.

87. Cahill, "Can Theology Have a Role in 'Public' Bioethical Discourse?" p. S14.

RONALD COLE-TURNER

Theological Interpretations of Biotechnology: Issues and Questions

It is often assumed that religion should have something to say, even if wholly negative, about biotechnology. But isn't it odd, to put it mildly, to think that millennia-old ideas will offer guidance to anyone in thinking about the emerging challenges raised by genetics and biotechnology? Nevertheless, when a new technique such as cloning is announced, religious opinions are sought immediately, if only to provide a dissenting voice for the sake of journalistic conflict.

Someday in the future, perhaps when human germ-line modification has been attempted, some reporter might ask a religious scholar: "And what does your religious tradition have to *learn* from this development?" The very notion that a religious tradition *can learn anything new*, least of all from technology, might strike some as surprising and others as offensive. Many view religious ideas as stuck in a time warp, perhaps profound for the first century or maybe the fifteenth but not for ours. And some religious scholars and theologians share this view: Theology is complete and can accept no revision or expansion.

But that view is a minority one and generally not persuasive to religious scholars and theologians, at least in mainstream Protestantism. Nevertheless, only a handful of theologians have taken up the distinctive challenges posed by the new biology and, in particular, by genetics and biotechnology, not just for pastoral care or for moral decision making but as *theological* challenges or provocation for new forms of theological thinking. Rarely have theologians asked what genetics means for their theology.

Of course, in taking up that task, we want to avoid going to the opposite extreme, translating ancient theological ideas so thoroughly into modern forms of thought that one can scarcely find the original. When that happens, we allow theology to sound like nothing but cultural analysis. Theology comes to the present with a rich set of ideas, traditionally expressed as doctrines, which are wholly revisable in the light of new insights but not reducible to them. Religious traditions are living traditions, growing and expanding, drawing from their intellectual context while daring to speak to it. Theologians have always understood this, and despite occasionally exaggerated claims of deference to ancient sources, they have undertaken the theological task as a dialogue between the text and context, between tradition and the modern world. Traditional wisdom speaks only when it listens, and it is in the correlating of classic and contemporary that theology has something to say. Our situation today is only different in that we live in a time of explosive growth of knowledge and technique. If theology wishes to speak to this context, to speak to biotechnology, it must first listen and then learn to correlate what it hears with what it knows. This implies no disrespect for religious tradition, unless one thinks that tradition is dead. Like a living organism, a living faith tradition interacts with its environment and thereby maintains its own true identity.

And so we ask: What can theology—in this case, Christian theology—learn from genetics and biotechnology? A few academic theologians have begun to consider this question, but their work to date is tentative and exploratory. My goal is to build on their work, to map out in survey fashion the key problems that arise when genetics and religion intersect, and to offer some suggestions and proposals. This essay is organized according to theological themes. That is, I do not address topics in genetics or biotechnology, such as germ-line modification, and then ask what religion has to say. Rather, I start with the classic doctrines of Christian theology, such as creation, and ask how genetics challenges or helps us revise and enrich these ideas. The design and organization, therefore, are theological, as if the intended reader were an academic theologian. But, in fact, I hope others will read the essay, including those with no interest or attachment to theology. Why? What value might nontheologians find here? Theology, I believe, can provoke rich and valuable dialogue when its questions and proposals are considered seriously by those who disagree with its assumptions and conclusions. It enriches and is enriched when it provokes disagreement, tough questions, and counterproposals, and when its own ideas come back to it in new and different forms.

Traditional theology, as developed by the major figures of the Western Christian tradition,[1] contains highly elaborate doctrines of God, creation, humanity, and of the relationships among them. In every age, the major Christian theologians have sought to make sense of these key doctrines in terms of the insights of their age. They drew freely upon contemporary insight, pressing it into service as a source of theological understanding, and rarely did they interpret biblical or traditional texts with the sort of literalism that emerged in some circles in twentieth-century Christianity. That is not to say that these theologians did not experience a conflict between tradition and the contemporary. Traditional doctrines, which were formed by prior interaction between scripture and the surrounding context, will inevitably be at odds with changing contexts. Such conflict became intense and public in the nineteenth century with the rise of Darwinian evolution.

Now at the beginning of a new century, we are attaining a highly sophisticated understanding of genes and the complexity of their functions. The rapid advance of scientific understanding in genetics and its explanatory power in other areas of biology, such as evolution, offers theology a rich and comprehensive explanatory context in which to expound its classic motifs. Core theological ideas about God, creation, human nature, and the human predicament, the goodness and the disorder of creation, and the future of creation are all affected by new perspectives, particularly the insights emerging from genetics research. I will consider these areas of doctrine and ask what new challenges and insights genetics and biotechnology might offer.

The discussion is organized in four parts. First, I ask what new knowledge arises from genetics that can lead to new theological understanding of God the creator. Second, what can genetics and biotechnology reveal to us about creation? Third, what can theology learn from genetics about human nature, and about freedom and moral responsibility? And fourth, I consider how biotechnology puts us human beings into a new situation vis-a-vis nature, calling for a new theological vision of the human role in nature.

Genetics and the Creator

Central to the understanding of God is the belief that God is the creator. This is the presupposition of all other theological beliefs, for God's power to renew and redeem is predicated upon God's prerogative as creator. According to the traditional doctrine, God brings the whole creation into existence, orders and sustains it, and draws it toward its final destiny. God is the Creator of all things visible and invisible, the source of both form and matter and that upon which all things depend for their being and order. In its relation to God, the creation is entirely good, containing no intrinsic conflict between good and evil. Evil and disorder arise, however, because creatures turn from God the supreme good to lesser goods, thereby confounding the moral order of the universe. This disordering act of will brings natural disorders as a fitting punishment. In its earliest form, Christian theology saw sickness and death (understood primarily as separation from God) as the result of rebellious will or sin. Redemption, centered for Christians in the death and resurrection of Jesus Christ, overcomes the destructive power of sin and death by incorporating its effects into the very being of God.

The divine act of creating must now be understood in light of cosmic and biological evolution. Through the various sciences, including genetics, we see complex processes such as random mutation and natural selection, understood more broadly as the interplay between chance and law-like regularities. The creation—this highly organized, complex, and cosmic and planetary system, including life on earth—is the result of the interplay between chance and regularity, and this interplay appears to be the working out, over time, of what is given in the origin of the universe. If the creation is the result of the dynamic interplay of these processes, then the divine act of creating must be understood as expressed through these intermediate processes.

Furthermore, it must be possible for theologians to imagine how this could be in a way that is consistent with the universe as we understand it through contemporary science. One way to do this is to propose that God determines the fundamental, law-like regularities that appear to be given or built into nature at the outset, regularities that define the processes by which the elaborate structures of creation are formed. Speaking of the source of the given, law-like regularities, Arthur Peacocke has made the helpful suggestion that "this givenness, for a theist, can only be regarded as an aspect of the God-endowed features of this world."[2] He continues: "Such potentialities a theist must regard as written into creation by the Creator's intention and purpose and must conceive as gradually being actualized by the operation of 'chance' stimulating their coming into existence."[3] In this way, theology understands God's role as the original determinations "which, as it were, 'load the dice' in favor of life and, once living organisms have appeared, also of increased complexity, awareness, consciousness and sensitivity, with all their consequences."[4] God can thus be understood as creative in bringing about those conditions upon which the emergence and evolution of life depends. In this view, God does not precisely design any species, much less any gene sequence or combination. But God will be seen as continuously creative in that the effects of God's original determination are continuously and pervasively present.

But does this view confine God's activity to establishing the initial conditions from which all else is derived? Does God not have an ongoing *direct* role to play, not merely working with and through intermediate processes, not merely watching what they might create, but acting directly upon them? Does God determine not only the original conditions but also discrete effects? For any proposal of this sort of direct divine action to have credibility, it must begin with our best understanding of these natural processes and then ask how God might be understood as acting directly within them, without thereby violating their integrity, which God, presumably, first established. Robert J. Russell has suggested that it may be fully consistent with our knowledge of quantum physics and genetics, and in particular with the largely unexplored connection between them, to see God as acting without interfering or violating the laws of nature. Russell argues that, consistent with science, God may be thought of as the sufficient explanation (but not a cause) of quantum events. God may be said to "act" in this way. But do quantum effects matter in the world of everyday experience? The ocean consists of quantum effects that appear not to affect navigation in the slightest. Do quantum events cancel out each other's effects at the level of ordinary experience? One way, Russell argues, for quantum effects to count in determining the phenomena of the life-size world of everyday experience is through genetics. Basic genetic processes of mutation and recombination, residing as they do at the level of molecule and atomic bond, may be thought of not as strictly random but as determined by events at the quantum level. By virtue of being the sufficient explanation of quantum events, Russell argues, God can therefore be said to act via genetic mutations to influence evolution.

> God shapes and guides biological evolution providentially by actions whose effects occur within the quantum mechanical processes underlying specific genetic mutations. . . . The effect of the acts of God in specific quantum events within the DNA molecule is to realize specific genetic mutations whose presence in the germ line, amplified by replication, and expression in the phenotype may bequeath to progeny potential adaptive advantage. In this way, and in others, God directs evolution toward God's purposes.[5]

Objections to Russell's proposal may be based on science, philosophy, and theology. Is his understanding of the relationship between quantum event and genetic event correct? Has he correctly interpreted the philosophical significance of quantum physics so as to allow, without contradiction from the science, the claim that God may be thought of as the sufficient explanation for such events? And has he implicated God too directly in the processes not just of evolution but of genetic disease, in effect demoting God to be merely a cause among causes, and the cause of evil at that?[6] For here we confront an obvious and classic problem, namely, how to make sense of God's responsibility for pain and suffering. If God is *directly* involved in such things as genetic mutations, it will be difficult if not impossible *not* to blame God for sickness. My own view is that even though quantum physics and genetics might permit theology to accept Russell's proposal, theology has other grounds for rejecting it because it too directly implicates God as the cause of pain.

The relationship between divine creativity and creaturely pain is not a new problem for theology nor is it raised for the first time by genetics, but genetics does reveal the intimate link between creativity (via mutations as the source of evolutionary novelty) and disease (mutations as genetic defects). This helps theology, I believe, to recognize that in the physical cosmos, with life having emerged according to these rules, there is simply no way to separate creativity from pain, or more precisely to separate some causes of creativity from some causes of suffering, namely genes. Eliminate the cause of pain and you eliminate the whole creation.

But of course we human beings do not experience nature as a whole process; we experience it in discrete sets of circumstances, some of which can be painful or lead to horrible suffering. We are not inclined to interpret the tragic events of our own lives as the necessary condition for the vast, evolutionary process. And so theology cannot be content merely with generalizations about nature *as a whole* but must say something about the specific set of circumstances that confront individuals. Christians have generally believed that certain conditions, such as that of an infant to be born to a brief life or a life of constant pain, are not what God intends for us. We acknowledge that we could not have this creation, as we now understand it, without its vulnerability to such things as cancer or genetic disease. But God the creator, intending to create through this process, does not intend every state or condition that arises in this process.

According to Arthur Peacocke, "In human life we must accept, for the stability of our own mental health and of our faith, that reality has a dimension of chance interwoven with a dimension of causality—and that through such interweaving we come to be here and new forms of existence can arise."[7] And elsewhere he comments:

> The chance disorganization of the growing human embryo that leads to the birth of a defective human being and the chance loss of control of cellular multiplication that appears as a cancerous tumour are individual and particular results of that same interplay of "chance" and "law" that enabled and enables life at all. . . . Even God cannot have one without the other.[8]

The view that emerges here for theology, in light of genetics, is that God takes great risks in creating. Evolutionary creativity depends upon mutations, but mutations lie at the basis of genetic disease, both inherited and acquired (as in the case of most cancers). A world without such disease would be a world without life itself. Or as John Polkinghorne observes:

> If love implies the acceptance of vulnerability by endowing the world with an independence which will find its way through the shuffling operations of chance rather than by rigid divine control . . . then the world that such a God creates will look very much like the one in which we live, not only in its beautiful structure but also in its evolutionary blind alleys and genetic malfunctions.[9]

In one sense, at least, the problem of suffering is shown to be a bogus problem, for it assumes a created world like this one, except that evil in the form of innocent suffering can be neatly eliminated without losing, not merely the value of learning from suffering, but life itself. For if mutations are necessary for life but lead inexorably to suffering, it is impossible to eliminate the one without destroying the other. Any hypothetical "perfect world" created in this way is a perversion of imagination, one that ideology does not have to explain away because it cannot exist in the first place. Now of course, contemporary theology has other things besides this to say about pain and suffering (largely by reversing the classic insistence that God does not suffer). But on the link between creativity and suffering, genetics helps theology find its way through false problems.

Indeed, God must be seen as a creator who explores the potentialities of the creation, who sets in motion processes that are *not* predetermined and whose outcome is unknown much less controlled even by God. God is a creator who has shared creativity with the creation, distributing the processes of creativity throughout the cosmic process. Theologians debate whether such a God is overly limited, or how these limits are to be understood. Is this a diminution of our concept of God, a whittling down of divinity to fit our worldview? Or is it a corrective to the theological excesses of earlier ages, when God was praised with superlatives such as infinite or unlimited? Might it not even be that God is best thought of as *self-limiting*, that is, a God who by creating shares power and prerogative with the creation? The theological debate over divine limits and self-limits began independent of theological attention to genetics. But the impact of genetics upon theology will be to encourage the view that God is limited, sharing power, as it were, with the creation.

Belief in a divine creator raises an additional set of questions upon which genetics and biotechnology have a bearing. We are now forced to ask new questions about the purpose of other species, the limits of the right of human beings to alter them, and the ownership of biological components. In framing its response, the Christian tradition is theocentric; that is to say, it insists that God is the center of value and that all things are to be valued in respect to their relationship to God, not to their usefulness to us. According to James Gustafson, a theocentric perspective reframes the usual contexts of value: "If one's basic theological perception is of a Deity who rules all of creation, and one's basic perception of life in history and nature is one of patterns of interdependence, then the good that God values must be more inclusive than one's normal perceptions of what is good for me, what is good for community, and even what is good for the human species."[10] But now, of course, *we* can create novel strains of animals (e.g., the oncomouse), define their purpose, and advertise their price. We can do this by directly manipulating the organism's DNA, which, more than any other physical component of an organism, defines its purpose or identity. It has been suggested that DNA constitutes the physical correlate to the Aristotelian *telos*, that inner principle of form and purpose that defines each thing. DNA is different and in many ways *less* than what Aristotle had in mind by *telos*, but when we redefine an organism's DNA we are surely putting our mark on its identity and purpose.

When, by genetic engineering, we modify a strain of mice to develop tumors, are we acting anthropocentrically? Have we put ourselves and not God at the center of the value definition for another species? Have we made them so that their entire existence revolves entirely around us and our purpose? This is the difference between biology and biotechnology: We are not merely naming what we find but making what we want. Of the oncomouse, we must ask whether, theologically considered, it should be the purpose of any species or any strain to *develop cancer on cue*. Is it the purpose of any species to be a model organism for disease? The question is posed here, not as one of animal welfare, but of a theocentric view of the world. What is the relationship between the animal and God? Is God's claim to define the organism consistent with our creating a disease model through gene knock-out technology? Personally, I believe a theocentric view can permit limited animal research, including the use of genetically engineered models. My point is that these new techniques challenge theology to rethink the meaning of God's relationship with all creatures and the right human interaction within that relationship. We need a theological rationale, on theocentric grounds, for genetic modification of other species.

When we lay claim through patent law to intellectual property protection for the exclusive use of our knowledge of living things and their component parts, are we claiming an additional privilege to exclude purposes inconsistent with our own, thus further defining ourselves as the center of value? Some see biological patenting as a direct challenge to the classic view that God is the sole owner of nature, especially of living things. It has been suggested that "as Creator, God has a kind of ownership right, not of exclusion or domination, but perhaps best understood as the right to define the purpose and value of each creature, as well as to define the right or moral relationship among creatures." In this view, nature "is not . . . utterly valueless except as raw material for human use, devoid of any worth except what we ascribe to it. Nature is value-laden not because we value it but because God does, and our valuing of nature must conform to God's."[11] Given the recent course of development taken by biotechnology, the question for theology is whether biological patents are appropriate expressions of human activity within a theocentric world. Some religious leaders oppose patenting because they believe it contributes to a reductionist attitude toward living things and toward their commodification. The notion of commodification, I believe, is best understood within the context of a theocentric worldview. Commodification is objectionable because it tends to define the value of creatures in terms of their usefulness to us and not their relationship to God. While I believe that biological patenting does *not* violate a theocentric view and that in fact it can be a legitimate mechanism for appropriate commercial activity in this arena, I agree with the religious critics of patenting that these are important concerns. The claim that gene patenting is merely a legal or economic issue is offensive to anyone who takes theocentrism seriously. As one who is theocentric but also open to patenting, I must be prepared to argue that patenting is the best (although not perfect) way to stimulate the research and development God intends.

Genetics and the Creation

Beyond all this, genetics and biotechnology offer rich suggestions about the creation itself. They offer new insight into the subtle complexities of the organic world. They prompt theology to recognize the unity of life at the molecular level and the proximity between *Homo sapiens* and other species, and they challenge traditional theological assertions about human uniqueness. But in two areas in particular, having to do with the problem of pain and with the unfinished nature of the creation, genetics and biotechnology offer especially helpful challenges to the doctrine of creation.

Christian theology portrays the creation as good and not as some conflicted mix of good and evil. Nevertheless, the good creation is deprived of its true, original integrity or goodness. This was expounded in the past through a doctrine of the fall and the curse of nature, according to which nature becomes less hospitable to human beings than it was originally to Adam and Eve. Classic Christian theologians held that there is an original or integral condition of creation that is marred as a result of sin, and so they attributed these creaturely imperfections to the effects of sin. In the writings of Francis Bacon, this doctrinal framework became the justification for technology, through which human beings repair nature and thereby restore their original relationship to nature.[12]

Centuries before genetics, these theologians spoke of nature, inheritance, defect, and disorder, all brought about by the fall. Even though genetics and evolution pull the narrative rug from beneath this classic explanation, the language of genetic defect or disorder remains in common secular discourse. An echo of this framework is still heard in phrases such as "remaking Eden"[13] and in the notion of genetic disease based on genetic defects, together with the justification for the development and use of technology to repair the "defect," if possible. Without the classic theological underpinnings, however, these echoes are vague legitimizations that merely justify technology without imposing limits upon it, for they cannot specify the original condition of the creation beyond which technology ought not aspire. Technology has no limit because evolution has no end. Even so, gene "therapy" or "repair" is widely supported while enhancement is generally viewed with suspicion, probably for reasons that are difficult to fathom because they lie deep in our religious pasts, where they are grounded in ghosts of doctrines no longer believed, at least in their original form.

With the synthesis of Darwinian evolution and genetics in twentieth-century biology, new perspectives on nature and a wholly new view of disease, "defect," and "disorder" have come into view. Notions of "defect" and "therapy," in spite of the fact that they are spoken of frequently in straightforward scientific reports, are in fact called into question for theologians as well as geneticists, by genetics itself. It is now clear that no clear, bright line separates good genes from defective genes, but that various alleles, together with variation in regulatory sequences or in interactive effects with other genes or with the environment, lead to a continuous spectrum of phenotypic expression. This is not to say that value categorizations are impossible, merely that they cannot be taken as simple or binary, as in good versus defective, but as poles on a spectrum.

Furthermore, it must now be seen that diversity found along this spectrum has *value in itself as a necessary precondition for evolution and for the robustness of ecosystems.* So the classic theological view of nature as good but fallen into disorder needs to be reconsidered. Nature, as God's creation, is good, and its diversity is a necessary component of its goodness. What we experience as "disorder" is not something nature has lapsed into but is a necessary part of its goodness of the whole.

Recently, some theologians have come to see creation not only as a dynamic process but as one that is as yet "unfinished." This is not to say that the creation is like Schubert's 8th, only half done, or that it is some ill-conceived project whose status cannot be measured because its meaning and destiny are being made up as it goes along. No, the creation is good and it is complete in its goodness and integrity. It is a complete system that is richly generative of more creativity and novelty, and its destiny is determined before it exists, in God's decision to create an *other* as a mirror of divine glory and as a counterpart to divine fellowship. Its purpose is established, and that is to generate expanded possibilities of praise and glorification of its creator. Nor should it be thought that the creator is egotistical, but simply that in praising its creator the creation transcends itself most gloriously in the wonder of what it can become as a community of ecstatic joy. Therefore, as a precisely defined totality, it is nevertheless unfinished, for God has determined that it remain constantly open in its capacity to generate new species, new structures, new capacities, and new thresholds of complexity.

Current research in genetics helps illumine this boundless creativity. Genetics discloses how a simple structure (DNA>>RNA>>Protein) yields endless variation. In particular, biotechnology itself must be seen as a newly emergent phenomenon of creation. It is itself one of the new capacities that have emerged, for although biotechnology uses natural processes such as restriction enzymes that have existed for aeons, their use by a conscious agent acting intentionally within a cultural framework is a novelty of epochal proportions. Here evolution has given rise not to a new species but to a whole new era in which one species begins to understand and order the processes by which it has come into existence.[14] The significance of this moment is easily overlooked or minimized because it is occurring in the blink of an eye, in the course of our own brief lifetimes.

We can now sum up various themes that have been considered. Theology, drawing on genetics and biotechnology, may now see more clearly than ever that creation is a continuously dynamic and emergent process, capable of generating new forms and levels of complex organization. We human beings ourselves are the result of these generative processes, and through us evolution has become conscious of itself, of the mechanisms upon which it rests, and of technologies through which these processes might be controlled. For theology, this entire emergent process, including now the human ability to understand and direct it, is the creation of God. Our task is to comprehend ourselves and our role within this comprehensive system, which embraces both creation and creator in mutual relationship. Theology may now understand creation in greater detail than ever before. But by understanding more completely, theology may then contextualize, relativize, and define technology, including biotechnology. Our human role as nature's engineers must be understood, theology insists, within the rubric of the prior claim that nature is God's creation, and our engineering must submit to God's right to define the creation and all its creatures. We will come to this theme in the section titled "The New Human Role in Nature." First, however, we consider a more troubling question, whether, now that we have the technical capacity to alter nature, we possess the moral and spiritual qualities to do so wisely, and what genetics itself can reveal to us about these qualities.

Human Nature and the Human Predicament

According to Christian theology's earliest anthropology, derived from Hebrew roots, human beings are biological organisms, made of dust. This organism is capable of the moral and spiritual life, but that capacity arises from the organic and does not require a separate, spiritual substance or ontologically distinct "soul," as dualism maintains. Of course, Christian theologians over the centuries have often espoused dualism, in large part because they were convinced that a physical or organicist view of human nature was unable to account for the religious or moral dimension of the person. They drew upon dualistic ideas from Greek or Enlightenment thinkers, which were widely accepted, and incorporated them into theology.

Today, mostly because of advances in neuroscience and genetics, we live amidst a conceptual revolution regarding our own human nature. At precisely the time when we are contemplating our own self-modification, we are learning to re-think the very meaning of our humanity. Neuroscience and brain imaging techniques offer concrete evidence of brain/mind relationships, and genetics offers tantalizing clues about the environmental and genetic determinants of human behavior and personality. Together, these fields of inquiry suggest that human beings are affected, in their core capacities and functions, by their evolutionary past, their genetic make-up, and their neurological development. The precursors of morality, social abilities, and thought itself are all products of this process.[15] This is not to suggest that our thoughts or acts are determined by our genes or by the evolutionary process, but that the fundamental capacities, such as the brain itself, emerge from this natural history and bear the legacies of its selective pressures.

Contemporary behavior genetics, together with neuroscience and related fields, provides evidence in favor of a unitary view of the human self.[16] These areas of science discredit dualism. But perhaps more important, they offer hints as to how a unified view of human nature is consistent with our having moral and spiritual capacities. Christianity, which has often wavered between dualism and psychosomatic unity, now has clear encouragement to support psychosomatic unity and thus good reason to go about reclaiming this element of its tradition and filling in the details in this traditional view. In doing so, theology should make it clear that it rejects both dualism and reductionism, and that a contemporary restatement of the human person as a psychosomatic unity is theologically and scientifically compelling. Theology may have an important public role to play in making a clear case for the human as a psychosomatic unity in the face of reductionist tendencies such as a genetic determinism, which now seem on the ascendancy in popular culture.

The view that is emerging from behavior genetics is that human life as we experience it in all its complexity arises from the life-long interplay of genes and environment. The role of genes in behavior is significant but subtle—significant in that the genes we inherit count substantially in explaining why we differ from other people, but subtle in that the mechanisms that connect genes to behavior are such that the contribution of any one gene is normally quite small. Thus far, behavior genetics suggests that human moral and intellectual capacities can be compromised easily by genetic problems. For example, the study of the family in the Netherlands in which half the men inherited a "knock-out" mutation on the X chromosome in the gene for monoamine oxidase A, an enzyme that breaks down serotonin, shows fairly dramatically that low intelligence, impulsivity, and violent behavior can result from a single base mutation.[17] We might expect to find other, similar examples of core neurological processes comprised by similar genetic mutations. While mental ability is the byproduct of many genes interacting with environmental factors, recent research suggests "that genetic enhancement of mental and cognitive attributes such as intelligence and memory in mammals is feasible,"[18] and that someday it may be possible to alter one or more genes, resulting in a significant gain in mental stability.

Although we often speak as if each gene were rigidly linked to a trait, we must remember that genes code for proteins, and this relationship itself is complicated by gene/gene interactions, by the effects of regulatory sequences, and by the environment. Furthermore, the gene-to-protein pathway merely begins what can be a highly complex, interacting cascade of events that may result in the trait clearly expressed, but may not, depending upon other factors impinging upon the pathway. In addition, we have to add the further complexities of development, in which genes switch on and off, or regulation, whereby noncoding regions determine the amount of gene product in ways that are absolutely critical to successful function; and of pleiotropic effects, whereby genes may play more than one role or bear on more than one trait.

Genetic and molecular pathways are complex at the cellular level, and so we must wonder whether we can ever hope to understand top-down effects from the psychological or personal level that impinge upon these cellular processes. Can the *person as person* act on the gene/protein/

cell system so that the person exerts causal influence on the system? Are our genes or our neurotransmitters responsible for our actions, or are *we*? Can it be said that in addition to all the molecular modifiers, there is a modifying effect that comes from *the person* or from *the soul*? Is there a role here for human freedom and responsibility?

Theology, of course, has always answered yes to these questions, but its answer has at times been compromised by its acceptance of dualism. A purported advantage of dualism is that the nonphysical soul is immune from mechanistic causation, and so the will (which resides in the soul) is wholly free of the impingement of the physical. Uncontrolled by the body or the brain, the will nevertheless somehow controls all things, like the pilot in the ship, acting but not being acted upon. But if theology today now rejects dualism, and if it seeks to learn from neuroscience and behavior genetics, then it will need a new definition of "soul," one that is not dualistic but is sufficiently clear and compelling to stand as a firewall against reductionism and genetic determinism. As tempting as it might be, theology cannot abandon the notion of soul. This old world, cleared of its dualistic interpretation, must now serve as a barrier against reductionism and genetic determinism.

Here is a proposed definition that seeks to avoid dualism and reductionism:

> According to traditional Christian theology, human beings are like other animals: we are made of the dust of the ground. But we are unlike all other animals in several important ways. Our mental capacities are far greater, our emotional sensitivities far more subtle, and our social relationships far richer and more complex than those of any other species. We alone have the capacity for spoken language, for moral awareness, for free moral choice, for creativity, and perhaps most importantly, for a relationship with God, a relationship that we believe will continue forever. These special capacities, taken together, are the human soul.[19]

V. Elving Anderson also suggests a "capacities" approach to the question of our core identity, and of course agrees that these central human capacities are genetically defined: "Our capacities for moral and spiritual activity are genetically conditioned, but our use of them remains a matter of personal choice."[20] This way of putting it, however, could be read as a form of latent or residual dualism, as if certain human capacities were genetically constrained but "personal choice" somehow remains immune from biological conditioning. Better to say that "personal choice" is one of the conditioned capacities, that in fact there is nothing about us, no metaphysically privileged inner core, that is free of the constraints of biological and genetic flaws.

In particular, we must insist that *the will itself*, or the capacity to define and direct the self, to understand the consequences of actions and to choose among them, is itself constrained by biological and genetic factors. As evidence, we can refer again to the study of the effects of the mutation in the monoamine oxidase A gene.[21] The capacities commonly understood as will are compromised by this mutation, suggesting that genetic and biological factors play a role, not just in the brains of the affected subjects in the study, but for all of us. Mutated or not, the monoamine oxidase A gene appears to play a role in the emergence of the will in a person. In its mutated form, sadly, we see unusual constraints upon the will. But those of us without this mutation are also constrained, even if not as tightly in this respect. For everyone, the capacity for moral deliberation and choice is a complex byproduct of gene/environment interactions the outcome of which both create and constrain this capacity.

We must say, at the risk of paradox, that gene/environment interactions both create and limit freedom. This idea of limited freedom is wholly consistent with traditional Christianity, which insists that each person is sufficiently free to be responsible but not to be perfect. That is to say, according to Christian theology, we are not radically free, as if our freedom resided in a soul that is metaphysically distinct from the body or from the sphere of causal mechanism, or as if the human will lacked its own internal predispositions or inclinations.

On the one hand, human capacities such as the will emerge from the interplay of genetic and other biological factors and so must be seen as constrained by those factors. But on the other hand, while constrained, these complex capacities nevertheless act in concert in ways that are not wholly controlled or predicted by their biological causes. In that sense they transcend their causes and become causal in their own right. Moral agency or will, for instance, is a complex capacity that arises from genetic and other biological factors, of course in relation to social and environmental factors. But having emerged in the life development of the normal human being, will acts as an agent in its own right, and for its action the agent is responsible. Nevertheless, the will's own structure and its actions are predisposed or pre-inclined by genetic or other factors. The will emerges as a structured or inclined capacity, a structured agent, not as neutral or uninfluenced by causal antecedents. That is not to say that these causal factors control the will or compel it to act in one way or another; for if that were true, it would not be will at all but mere mechanism that directs human behavior, and we would not be responsible for our actions. Avoiding such a mechanistic view, we should say instead that causal factors such as genes, while not acting *on* the will, act to structure the will's own capacity for free action and free expression.

Genetics is particularly important for theology precisely in this regard, because from the field of genetics we can see how genes may bring about tendencies of the will, such as traits of personality or mood. These tendencies or traits do not act by external compulsion but by inner impulse that is subjectively indistinguishable from the will's own free choice. We can then speak of such things as a genetic susceptibility to a particular addiction, acknowledging the force of the susceptibility without conceding that there is no freedom. This view of the predisposed, constrained, and limited will is consistent with classic perspectives in Christian anthropology. Genetics, however, makes it possible for theology to clarify and elaborate this view as never before.

Furthermore, genetics lends added meaning and credibility to traditional Christianity's conviction that human beings are essentially naïve, superficial, and self-deceived. We tend to see ourselves as inherently simple, morally linear, and usually clear-headed when in fact we are confused and full of inner conflicts, willing one thing and its opposite at one and the same time and with a single but muddled will. Thinkers as different as Augustine and Freud have offered their analyses, but genetics now offers clear evidence that human persons are complex, multifactorial, and conditioned by processes that are not fully understood at the level of their own consciousness. We are an enigma to ourselves, as Augustine would say, and that in part because we are constrained by genetic and biological factors that condition consciousness and agency.

If classic theology makes any prediction here, it is that as we learn bits and pieces of the genetics of complex human capacities and as gene/behavior pathways are elucidated, we will latch on to these explanations of behavior as excuses or as simplistic causal mechanisms, once again thinking that we see ourselves more clearly than we really do. Indeed, as we now attain a complete knowledge of the human genome and enter into the era of human functional genomics, we will begin to contemplate the totality of genetic factors to the extent that they define not just health but our whole being. Will we not then be tempted to act on ourselves or on our progeny, as if we could improve *persons* with a simple pharmacological or genetic alteration? Now, we must avoid dualism precisely at this point. We must not say that pharmacological (Prozac or Ritalin) or genetic alteration does *not* alter the soul or the core capacities that define the person. We must even concede that these alterations clearly improve the functioning of some capacities. Ritalin, for instance, seems to give coherence and a personal, moral focus to some people diagnosed with attention deficit disorder. But precisely because of the clarity and power of such interventions and of our growing knowledge on which they are based, we must (theology would urge) refuse to exaggerate our clarity or think that we are now transparent to ourselves. If reductionism were true, we would in time become transparent to ourselves, at least in respect to gene/trait relationships. But according to Christianity, we are *inherently and forever enigmatic* precisely because we are psychosomatic unities with selves that transcend our genes and our knowledge of them.

In one very important respect, genetics contributes something radically new to Christian theology. Remembering that genetics is the study of differences, we must ask what we should make of differences among human beings in the precise shape of the genetic constraints of these capacities. "We have only a limited appreciation, however, of the extent of individual diversity in these capacities."[22] Traditional theology tended to see all human beings as more or less equal in their moral or spiritual state. Human wills were seen as equally inclined away from the perfect life. Now, however, we see quite a different picture. Indeed, we are only now on the threshold of momentous discoveries in behavior genetics, and increasingly it will become clear how we human beings differ from each other in subtle but sometimes profound ways. For theology, this will mean that forms of healing and grace will also take individual contours.

An issue of great significance for science policy is the question of the status of the embryo. The view that the embryo is a person at conception is relatively new in Christian theology. From its beginning, Christian ethics has most often regarded abortion as unacceptable (at least for all but the most extreme circumstances), but the status of embryonic and fetal life was not a subject for doctrinal clarity. Only in recent years has anti-abortion conviction combined with biological understandings of conception and embryonic development to lead to the conclusion, held at the very least by a vocal minority, that an embryo is a person. The impact of this view on science policy is felt, for instance, in areas such as human stem cell research. The view is not essential to Christianity nor is it supported by many theologians.

Theologians who hold alternative views of human personhood and its emergence during fetal development should try to make their views more clear and convincing to wider audiences.

The New Human Role in Nature

The rapid growth of knowledge in genetics is accompanied by the growing power and precision of the technologies of gene manipulation that already make it possible for us to modify organisms to suit human specifications. Theology can learn from the science of genetics, but it must also take notice of the simple fact that through biotechnology human beings are now casting themselves in a radically new role in nature, as its engineers at the level of DNA sequences and genomes.

Christian theology tends to endorse this activist, engineering relationship with nature. The classic perspective is grounded in the mandate found in Genesis 1-2: Human beings are to have dominion over the earth and other creatures, to name them (i.e., to know and define their essence), and to till and keep the earth, tending the garden. Historically these texts have been summarized by the term "stewardship," which claims that human beings are God's stewards, exercising a limited authority to care for and use the creation, but always under the claims of God. Alongside stewardship is the notion that human beings are created in the image of God, as God's assistants or viceroys, as bearers of the divine quality of rationality, and as existing in relationship or community. With these themes, Christianity has encouraged the study and the reordering of nature. As we noted earlier, the doctrine of the fall plays an important role here, for it provides a way to say that creation is good and yet needs repair or therapy, including gene therapy.

But now, because of the growing power of biotechnology, these traditional notions are inadequate depictions of our present role. Not only has technology grown in power, but also our fundamental assumptions about nature and creation have changed from a static system with fixed species to a dynamic system with constantly emerging novelty. So now we must ask how human beings, armed with genetic engineering, should be understood as playing a role in God's ongoing creative relationship with nature. To replace older terms such as steward or gardener, some theologians have proposed the term "co-creator." Philip Hefner has coined the phrase "created co-creator" in order to stress that while we possess creative powers, we are forever creatures, part of the fabric of the creation.

Human beings are God's created co-creators whose purpose is to be the agency, acting in freedom, to birth the future of what is most wholesome for the nature that has birthed us—the nature that is not only our own genetic heritage, but also the entire human community and the evolutionary and ecological reality in which and to which we belong. Exercising this agency is said to be God's will for humans.[23]

Sometimes the phrase "playing God" is also used to describe the human role. Most often this is used pejoratively, the most famous example being Paul Ramsey's remark that "Men ought not to play God before they learn to be men, and after they have learned to be men they will not play God."[24] Allen Verhey has offered the helpful suggestion that "playing God" is not necessarily a bad term but can be used if we are mindful of the exacting conditions, morally, of what it means to act as God acts, in compassion and for justice.[25] Ted Peters links "playing God" with "image of God" and suggests that "we should play human in the *imago Dei* sense—that is, we should understand ourselves as created co-creators and press our scientific and technological creativity into the service of neighbor love, of beneficence."[26]

Can biotechnology really be dignified with such theological labels as "co-creation"? What criteria would have to be met to deserve this status? Surely the technology would have to have sufficient power to make a difference in the outcome of the evolutionary process of creation. Biotechnology seems to be well on the way to meeting that criterion. But we must have some idea of what God is doing in the creation, what God's purposes are, and what role we can play in helping to achieve them. Such a consciousness, if possible at all, must be so shaped in human consciousness that we can confidently exercise our technological gifts toward God's intended end. What is God's future for the creation? Without some guiding vision operationalized in technology objectives, we cannot yet claim that we are co-creators. The challenge facing theology here is twofold: first, to create vivid and visionary metaphors of human action in faithful relation to the broadest possible contexts of meaning and ultimacy; and second, to make these metaphors effective in concrete human action so that they actually guide our collective behavior.

With stem cell technology, somatic cell nuclear transfer (for reproductive and nonreproductive purposes), and human germ-line modification all on the near horizon of the future, the need for compelling and effective visions is urgent. Often we try to draw a line between therapy and enhancement, assuming that therapy helps people live normal human lives but enhancement is an irresponsible escape from normalcy, with dangerous social implications. But it is increasingly recognized that it is impossible to draw a clear and enforceable line between therapy and enhancement, or to say that we will develop techniques for therapy but not allow their use for enhancement.[27] To be honest, we have to recognize that Western religion and culture have always endorsed many forms of personal enhancement (or salvation) as not merely optional but mandatory. According to Dean Hamer, "we soon will have the ability to change and manipulate human behavior through genetics."[28] If we should modify our behavior by traditional means of education or religious discipline, why not through genetics?

Where are we going, and how far will we go? Are we now "co-creators" of our own creatureliness? Are we becoming partly *self-created co-creators*? Will we transcend our own species and become *post-human*? Consider the comments of Lee Silver. Referring to a time about two centuries from now, he writes:

> It was a critical turning point in the evolution of life in the universe. . . . Throughout it all, there were those who said we couldn't go any further, that there were limits to mental capacity and technological advances. But those prophesied limits were swept aside, one after another, as intelligence, knowledge, and technological power continued to rise.[29]

For Silver, today's technology makes tomorrow's possible, not just in the trivial sense that one breakthrough builds on previous achievements, but that soon we will be able to engineer better engineers. Human beings will not only affect their own evolution, but in doing so, will put the whole process in overdrive. Silver continues, now referring to a time more than a millennium away:

> A special point has now been reached in the distant future. And in this era, there exists a special group of mental beings. Although these beings can trace their ancestry back directly to *homo sapiens*, they are as different from humans as humans are from the primitive worms with tiny brains that first crawled along the earth's surface.[30]

Granted, Silver's projections are exaggerated, especially in their time frame. But the underlying issue, that of any degree of human species self-transcendence, has now become an inescapable issue for all humanity and in particular for theology. Should we deliberately enhance our offspring to the point where they, or their descendants, are no longer exactly human? Will they be better off or much worse for our tinkering? Will they somehow become *more* human, more intelligent, more just, more loving, more creative, and more free than their creators? Will they become, as Silver suggests, better at engineering? Or will we have replaced ourselves through a perversion of procreation with mere artifacts, mere projections of our will who have no will themselves? Hans Jonas warned of any technological gamble that wagers the human present on the trans-human future:

> Now, this innate sufficiency of human nature, which we must posit as the enabling premise for any creative steering of destiny, and which is nothing other than the sufficiency (albeit fallible) for truth, valuation, and freedom, is a thing unique and stupendous to behold in the stream of becoming, out of which it emerged, which in essence it transcends, but by it can also be swallowed again. . . . Most evidently, the authority which it imparts can never include the disfiguring, endangering, or refashioning of itself. No gain is worth this price, no hope of gain justifies this risk.[31]

Proper reverence for the processes of creation that brought us forth, demands that we keep technology away from altering our own nature.

Theology has two responses to make, one fairly clear, and the other ambivalent and open-ended. First, theology must reject here any notion that nature, including now human nature, is mere raw material open to ceaseless human manipulation. Philip Hefner warns us of the danger of the prevailing worldview, according to which

> all of nature should finally be re-shaped in the ways that humans deem most desirable. . . . This is the major characteristic of the ideological garments in which genetic testing meets us. We approach nature—including our own human nature—in terms of what we can make of it; nature is not something we accept, rather it is the object of our fantastic ability to reshape the world.[32]

If such a worldview defines our genetic alteration of our offspring, then they, too, will become raw material for our overweening technological will. They will become mere artifacts, the ultimate projections of our drive to control all nature. Against this tendency to view nature as raw material, Christianity asserts its theocentric view that God, not human beings, defines the order and value of all creation and all creatures. For those committed to a theocentric view, any modification, any reordering, any engineering must conform to God's purpose.

But for this very reason, secondly, theology must be open to the possibility of human transcendence. To be theocentric is precisely to recognize that human survival, even that of the human species, is not the highest value in the cosmos, and that we may therefore consent to our own demise, to our becoming merely a transitional form along a divinely intended pathway toward the full realization of nature's potential. Theologians as far back as Irenaeus (c. 130–202) have understood human nature as partially complete and destined to full maturity that transcends the past or the present. Might we say that we now stand on the threshold of a human self-abrogation more profound than any religiously motivated act of self-denial, and that we are about to engineer deliberately our own incremental metamorphoses? Such a thought is at once terrifying and yet surprisingly appealing theologically, that we would sacrifice ourselves as a species in order to have a hand in creating a new species, a new humanity. Then we will have discovered a new civilization of advanced beings, not through space travel, but here in our progeny enhanced by our technology. Is this God's intention for life on earth? I am not suggesting that theology's answer is yes, or that our commitment to a theocentric view calls for our willingness to become a transitional form, even less at our own hands. I am simply trying to show that the stakes are very high and that biotechnology calls forth from theology, and from all of its secular alternatives, the most profound engagement.

NOTES

1. I have in mind here thinkers like Origen, Augustine, Aquinas, Martin Luther, John Calvin, Friedrich Schleiermacher, and in our own century, Karl Rahner, Karl Barth, Paul Tillich, Jurgen Moltmann, and Wolfhart Pennenberg.

2. Arthur Peacocke, *Theology for a Scientific Age: Being and Becoming— Natural, Divine and Human* (Minneapolis, Minn.: Fortress Press, 1993), p. 177.

3. Peacocke, *Theology for a Scientific Age*, p. 199. See also Arthur Peacocke, *God and the New Biology* (London: Dent, 1986), p. 97.

4. Peacocke, *Theology for a Scientific Age*, p. 199. See also Peacocke, *God and the New Biology*, p. 97.

5. Robert John Russell, "Does 'The God Who Acts' Really Act? New Approaches to Divine Action in Light of Science," *Theology Today* 54 (1997): 43–65, at 60. For an elaboration of the argument, see Robert John Russell, "Special Providence and Genetic Mutation," in *Evolution and Molecular Biology: Scientific Perspectives on Divine Action*, ed. R. J. Russell, N. Murphy, and F. Ayala (Notre Dame, Ind.: University of Notre Dame Press, 1998), pp. 191–223.

6. Ronald Cole-Turner and Brent Waters, *Pastoral Genetics: Theology and Care at the Beginning of Life* (Cleveland, Ohio: Pilgrim Press, 1996), pp. 88–92.

7. Peacocke, *God and the New Biology*, p. 99.

8. Peacocke, *Theology for a Scientific Age*, p. 126.

9. John C. Polkinghorne, *One World* (Princeton, N.J.: Princeton University Press, 1986), p. 67.

10. James M. Gustafson, *Theology and Ethics*, vol. 1 of *Ethics from a Theocentric Perspective* (Chicago: University of Chicago Press, 1981), p. 96.

11. Ronald Cole-Turner, "Theological Perspectives on the Status of DNA: A Contribution to the Debate over Genetic Patenting," in *Perspectives on Genetic Patenting: Religion, Science, and Industry in Dialogue*, ed. Audrey Chapman (Washington: American Association for the Advancement of Science, 1999), pp. 149–165, at 155.

12. David F. Noble, *The Religion of Technology: The Divinity of Man and the Spirit of Invention* (New York: Alfred A. Knopf, 1997).

13. Lee M. Silver, *Remaking Eden: How Genetic Engineering and Cloning Will Transform the American Family* (New York: Avon Books, 1997, 1998).

14. Ronald Cole-Turner, *The New Genesis: Theology and the Genetic Revolution* (Louisville, Ky.: Westminster/John Knox Press, 1993), pp. 42–47.

15. J. Wentzel Van Huyssteen, *The Shaping of Rationality: Toward Interdisciplinarity in Theology and Science* (Grand Rapids, Mich.: W.B. Eerdmans Publishing Co., 1999); Holmes Rolston, III, *Genes, Genesis, and God: Values and Their Origins in Natural and Human History*, The Gifford Lectures, 1997–1998 (Cambridge: Cambridge University Press, 1999).

16. For a summary of recent behavior genetics, see Dean Hamer and Peter Copeland, *Living with Our Genes: Why They Matter More Than You Think* (New York: Doubleday, 1998). For an attempt to interpret these findings within the context of Christianity, see Malcolm Jeeves, *Human Nature at the Millennium: Reflections on the Integration of Psychology and Christianity* (Grand Rapids, Mich.: Baker Books, 1997), pp. 83–97; V. Elving Anderson, "A Genetic View of Human Nature," in *Whatever Happened to the Soul? Scientific and Theological Portraits of Human Nature*, ed. Warren S. Brown, Nancey Murphy, and H. Newton Maloney (Minneapolis, Minn.: Fortress Press, 1998), pp. 49–72.

17. Brunner, H. G., M. Nelen, X. O. Breakefield, H. H. Ropers, and B. A. von Oost, "Abnormal Behavior Associated with a Point Mutation in the Structural Gene for Monoamine Oxidase A," *Science* 262 (1993): 578–80.

18. Y-P. Tang, E. Shimizu, G. Dube, C. Rampon, G. Kerchner, M. Zhuo, G. Lui, and J. Txien, "Genetic Enhancement of Learning and Memory in Mice," *Nature* 401 (1999): 63–69, at 63.

19. Ronald Cole-Turner, "Human Nature as Seen by Science and Faith," in *In Whose Image: Faith, Science, and the New Genetics*, ed. John P. Burgess (Louisville, Ky.: Geneva Press, 1998), pp. 121–132, at 123.

20. V. Elving Anderson, "A Genetic View of Human Nature," p. 71.

21. Brunner, H. G., "Abnormal Behavior," pp. 578–80.

22. V. Elving Anderson, "A Genetic View of Human Nature," p. 71.

23. Philip Hefner, *The Human Factor: Evolution, Culture, and Religion* (Minneapolis, Minn.: Fortress Press, 1993), p. 27.

24. Paul Ramsey, *Fabricated Man: The Ethics of Genetic Control* (New Haven, Conn.: Yale University Press, 1970), p. 138.

25. Allen D. Verhey, "Playing God," in *The Center for Bioethics and Human Dignity presents Genetic Ethics: Do the Ends Justify the Genes?* ed. John F. Kilner, Rebecca D. Pentz, and Frank E. Young (Carlisle [England]: Paternoster Press; Grand Rapids, Mich.: W. B. Eerdmans, 1997), pp. 60–74, at p. 61.

26. Ted Peters, *Playing God? Genetic Determinism and Human Freedom* (New York: Routledge, 1997), p. 15.

27. Erik Parens, ed., *Enhancing Human Traits: Ethical and Social Implications* (Washington: Georgetown University Press, 1998).

28. Hamer and Copeland, *Living with Our Genes*, p. 301.

29. Silver, *Remaking Eden*, pp. 292–93.

30. Silver, *Remaking Eden*, pp. 292–93.

31. Hans Jonas, *The Imperative of Responsibility: In Search of an Ethics for the Technological Age* (Chicago: University of Chicago Press, 1984), p. 33.

32. Philip Hefner, "The Genetic 'Fix': Challenges to Christian Faith and Community," in *Genetic Testing and Screening*, ed. Roger A. Willer, pp. 73–93, at 76.

Gerald P. McKenny

Religion, Biotechnology, and the Integrity of Nature: A Critical Examination

Does biotechnology, with its relentless reordering and commodifying of living things, violate the integrity of nature or life? On the basis of uncharacteristic but highly publicized expressions of opposition on the part of some religious leaders to practices such as the patenting of genes or the possibility of human germ-line gene therapy, one might assume that conflicts between religion and biotechnology arise because religious communities and scientists adhere to radically different views of the nature of life: that theological interpretations attribute a symbolic or sacred value, say, to DNA while scientists view it as mere matter, infinitely open to manipulation and commercialization by those capable of exploiting its secrets and harnessing its potential.[1]

So one might assume. But one would be at best only partially right. First, among "mainstream" religious bodies strong objections to biotechnology in principle are rare, in part because these bodies, who are most likely to weigh in on issues of biotechnology in a public way, generally support the aims of biotechnology. With one important exception (a report by a body of the World Council of Churches published in 1989), the criticisms of biotechnology in the official or quasi-official statements of such groups are restrained, and even when these criticisms take on a sharper edge, as they do in the exceptional case just mentioned, they are nevertheless carefully balanced by expressions of support in principle for agricultural and medical biotechnology.[2] Second, as we will see shortly, not all religious perspectives attribute a sacred or symbolic value to DNA, while some scientific perspectives ineluctably do.[3]

The general acceptance of biotechnology in principle should not lead us to conclude that there are no grounds for conflicts between religion and biotechnology in its particular instantiations or even to its approaches to nature or life in general. Ecclesial pronouncements on biotechnology often refer both to the potential risk of harmful consequences of actual or potential biotechnological developments and to matters of distributive justice and discrimination as morally relevant features of these developments. While the concerns expressed under these headings generally track those expressed by secular bioethicists, it would be wrong to conclude that they are, for that reason, less authentically religious concerns: It is as mistaken to expect that religious convictions will always entail views of the balance of goods and harms or the requirements of justice that differ substantially from those of others as it is to expect that these views will never differ. Other potential conflicts are more characteristic of, although not unique to or universal among, religious groups. Such conflicts may, for example, involve the status of human embryos. They may also involve what I explore here under the heading of the integrity of nature or of life.

By integrity of nature or life I mean to identify a fairly widespread if seldom scrutinized worry that at least some biotechnological developments or, at some level, all such developments, involve an illicit or at least highly suspect tampering with nature or life. This worry appears in two different forms in a number of ecclesial pronouncements on biotechnology. In what follows, I identify these two different forms, examine their implications, criticize them, and propose an alternative that I believe should command more attention among religious communities. Before proceeding, however, I must introduce several caveats and qualifications. First, worries about tampering with nature or life are not always a major concern in ecclesial statements and are often not made explicit. I highlight them here not because I think they are always the foremost concern of a religious community (though sometimes they are) but because I think they constitute a potential cause of genuine conflict between religion and biotechnology.[4] Indeed, while I cannot prove it here, I believe that the highly publicized objection of certain religious spokespersons to the patenting of genes ultimately follows from the kinds of concerns about nature and life I explore here. Second, this investigation is limited to pronouncements from Christian groups. This limitation does not deny the possibility of related worries among groups as diverse as orthodox Jews and deep ecologists. Third, my sources are primarily ecclesial statements rather than individual theologians. This presents the problem of how to determine for whom such statements speak. Official Catholic statements clearly reflect magisterial views, but one cannot always assume that the latter are widely shared among theologians or laypersons. Protestant and ecumenical statements lay no claims to magisterial authority, often reflect tensions and compromises among diverse interests in the ecclesial communions that sponsor them, are frequently the compilation of several authors with varying degrees of coordination, and are issued to an uncertain reception among their constituents. My interest, however, is not the question of what conflicts *are likely in fact to arise* between these communities and the biotechnology industry (a question for the sociology of religion), but rather the question of *whether there are grounds in the religious convictions themselves* for any such conflicts (a question of theological ethics), and if so, whether these religious convictions are the most appropriate way for religious groups to address what is at stake for their traditions in biotechnology. Finally, in what follows I range rather freely across diverse ecclesial statements. I consider myself justified in so doing in large part because, as will be evident shortly, I believe that the best way to understand worries about tampering with nature is to show how they follow from quasi-transcendental concepts that are never fully represented in any of the statements individually but which account for certain characteristics of these statements that are otherwise difficult to account for. I trust that the reader will see the value of this approach, although it neither precludes nor discounts efforts to understand the statements individually.

"Nature" and "Life Itself"

Claims about the ethical significance of the integrity of nature take a variety of forms in debates over biotechnology. For several reasons, such claims often fail to hold up under philosophical scrutiny. In some cases these claims turn out to be disguised concerns about other matters, in other cases they lead to conclusions most people find counterintuitive if they are applied consistently, while in yet other cases they apply equally to controversial forms of knowledge and technology and to those that almost everyone already accepts in principle. I will not pursue these potential criticisms here.[5] Instead, I will show how claims regarding the integrity of nature and the potential threats to the latter posed by certain developments in biotechnology follow from mutually incompatible quasi-transcendental concepts of life. These concepts are quasi-transcendental in the sense that they make possible certain ways of understanding life. As quasi-transcendental, these concepts need not be, and in the case of the ecclesial statements generally are not, thematized; rather, they form a framework that determines which characteristics of living things are deemed central or marginal; how living things are related to each other, to the nonliving, and to practices of knowing and intervening; and what ethical issues knowledge and intervention raise. In the case of ecclesial statements on biotechnology, two such concepts determine how life is understood and, in consequence, what is ethically at stake in intervening into living things. Once we identify these concepts and clarify their role, we not only will understand how their confusion generates certain inconsistencies in some of the statements, but will also discover that ecclesial statements that appear to be concerned with the same issues with regard to biotechnology—human dignity, reductionism, and the integrity of nature or the body—are in fact often concerned about very different things.

The first of these concepts I will refer to as "nature." I intend this term in a technical sense that implies an ontology consisting of some or all of the following kinds of orderings of living things: a taxonomic ordering that classifies life forms into distinct species; an ordering of parts, functions, or capacities to each other and to the whole; an ordering of living things to their perfection of form; and the rank ordering of species according to their proximity to the divine.[6] The essence of nature is order: In contrast to what the second concept will affirm, DNA has no special status in defining human nature or identity. Since the nonliving world also exhibits a kind of order, the distinction between the living and the nonliving, while by no means irrelevant, does not possess the significance that will be given to it by the second concept. Insofar as order is given normative significance, it follows that interventions at the level of molecular genetics are in principle permissible so long as they do not violate or circumvent natural order, however the latter is conceived. They may, of course, be morally wrong or problematic for various other reasons—the ordering of nature is not the only right- or wrong-making feature in most moral frameworks that recognize its importance—but in contrast to the second concept, the altering of nature is not itself a morally problematic issue, even when such alteration is extensive. While this view can be found among some Protestants and even among secular thinkers (e.g., Leon Kass in his emphasis on the primacy of form in characterizing human nature),[7] it is especially prominent in Roman Catholicism.

The success of evolutionary theory indicates the triumph of a second quasi-transcendental concept of the living as "life itself."[8] The concept of life itself governs many Protestant and (Protestant-dominated) ecumenical statements on genetic science and technology, although we will see that the adherence to this concept is incomplete. In contrast to nature as the ordering within or among living beings, life itself, as Sarah Franklin points out, is characterized by various features: metabolism; capacities for movement, growth, and reproduction; and the mechanisms of hereditary reproduction and evolution.[9] All of these features entail a much sharper distinction between the living and the nonliving, which now takes on a significance it could not have had under the aegis of order—a significance that persists despite the inability of the biological sciences to arrive at a precise concept of life. While particular conceptions of life itself may be formed by emphasizing any one of these features (as, for example, Hans Jonas's conception of life emphasizes metabolism),[10] three important characteristics of life—the interconnectedness of all living things, evolutionary change, and self-reproduction through the biogenetic mechanism of heredity—imply DNA or the genetic code as the essence of life and evolutionary and genetic factors as the key to what distinguishes life from nonlife.[11]

From this latter perspective, which governs many ecclesial statements, molecular genetic knowledge and intervention raise a different set of ethical issues. First, the increased significance of the distinction between life and nonlife, combined with the inability of the life sciences to secure the concept of life against its opposite, generates anxious efforts to distinguish between the natural and the artificial, to proclaim the superiority of the former over the latter, and to police against encroachments by the latter into the former. Nature is ethically significant, then, not in respect of its ordering but in respect of its naturalness, that is, its difference from what is made. The givenness of life—not a static or fixed givenness, but rather the dynamism of metabolic, developmental, or evolutionary processes—has a normative force against which disruptions of the given must justify themselves. From this perspective, intervention itself—not the violation of a natural order—is ethically charged even when, as in all major ecclesial statements, intervention is considered permissible in principle. Second, because all living beings are interconnected through their DNA and the evolutionary process, distinctions between species are less pronounced, and sharp distinctions between human beings and other species—not to mention the special role of human beings in virtually all pre-Darwinian thought—become difficult to maintain. This generates apparently opposite tendencies: one is the effort to expand the realm of moral considerability beyond humans to take in all living things; the other is the effort to reformulate notions of human dignity that depend on human distinctiveness from or transcendence of the rest of nature. As for the latter effort, if DNA, and not the status of humans in a natural order, is the essence of the human as living, human distinctiveness is more a matter of degree (and rather minimal degree at that), than of kind, and humans are subject to the same forces and dynamics that govern the rest of the living world. While this fact does not necessarily rule out a naturalistic conception of human dignity, it does limit the range of forms such a conception can take. Finally, the view of the gene as the essence of life enmeshes the concept of life itself in a doubly paradoxical relationship between mechanism and vitalism. First, while the genetic understanding of life secures the triumph of the explanation of life in mechanistic terms, the very success of this triumph seems to reduce life to the nonliving and thus imperils the adequacy of the mechanistic explanation itself as a concept of *life*.[12] This paradox keeps the ground fertile for new growths of vitalism. Second, as Franklin points out, mechanistic explanations, such as those of Richard Dawkins, which posit genes as selfishly reproducing, autotelic entities, perpetuate the very concepts such explanations were designed to overcome.[13] Franklin notes in this connection the similarity of the views of Dawkins and others to Aristotelian vitalism; perhaps more striking is that the portrait, drawn by Dawkins and others, of potentially immortal gene lineages using mortal organisms as ephemeral vehicles of self-perpetuation also recalls the classical concept of the immortal soul inhabiting a succession of bodies. The result of this double paradox is that while life itself is the quasi-transcendental ground of the modern biological sciences, the physical and biochemical methods of those sciences reduce life to the nonliving, and yet in this very process invite back, whether intentionally or not, the concepts of vitality and soul that these methods were concerned to expel in the first place. This vacillation between mechanism and vitalism is often portrayed as an irrational survival of an outmoded vitalistic biology among those who cannot accept the mechanistic implications of evolutionary and molecular biology, but there are good reasons to believe that such a vacillation is inevitable given the identification of a molecule as the essence of life itself. In any case, this vacillation ensures that DNA will be capable of signifying both the mechanistic reduction of living wholes (organisms) to interchangeable parts and the sacredness of life that resists, morally and spiritually if not scientifically and technologically, this reduction.[14]

Biotechnology and the Integrity of Nature in Catholic Ecclesial Statements

Once we have become clear about these two concepts, we are able to account for important differences among Catholic statements on the one hand and Protestant or ecumenical statements on the other hand, and to identify other differences in what appear to be similarities. One of the most striking features of many Catholic statements is how little importance they give to DNA in defining human nature. Official or quasi-official statements, including two influential declarations by Pope John Paul II, consistently define the essence of human nature not in genetic terms but in language made familiar by the Vatican II document *Gaudium et Spes*, for which union of body and soul (*corpore et anima unus*) is what is essentially human. One such statement, a report by a Working Party convened under the authority of The Catholic Bishops' Joint Committee on Bioethical Issues (U.K.) (hereafter CBJC), explicitly rejects the view that our genes have a privileged role in constituting human nature or personal identity. In opposition to some who oppose human germ-line gene therapy in principle on grounds of the centrality of the genome to human identity or development, the report argues that the genome is neither central to the identity of a person nor is it morally untouchable due to its role in human development. Rather, "the genome is simply one highly influential part of our bodies"; like other parts, it "may *in principle* be altered, to cure some defect of the body."[15] Since it is the unity of the person as body and soul, and not the givenness of one's genome, that is the essentially human, germ-line interventions are in principle permissible insofar as they do not violate this ordering of human nature (although in the view of the report, they may be, and under present technology and methods would be, impermissible for various other reasons, including the use of *in vitro* fertilization and the destruction of embryos).

In both the papal declarations and the CBJC report, the senses in which genetic interventions are potentially reductionistic and threatening to human dignity follow quite readily from this understanding of the essentially or characteristically human. In the papal declarations (and to a large extent in the CBJC report), dignity includes three components: respect for life, union of body and soul, and liberty.[16] The first component is respect for life, which entails the right to life "from the moment of conception to death" and status as an end and not a mere means to the collective good. This rules out genetic interventions that destroy embryos or subject them to experimentation. And (more relevant to our concerns), should they ever become possible, it rules out "manipulations tending to modify the genetic store and to create groups of different people, at the risk of provoking fresh marginalizations in society." In the latter case, however, it is unclear whether the "fresh marginalizations" would result from "groups of different people" who are superior to us, inferior to us, or both.[17] The second component rules out genetic interventions that might make use of forms of reproduction that separate the procreative act from the biological and spiritual union of husband and wife (e.g., artificial insemination and *in vitro* fertilization). It also rules out interventions that would distort or destroy the integral unity of body and soul, although it is unclear what kinds of interventions the pope has in mind here. Finally, liberty is violated when a genetic intervention "reduces life to an object, when it forgets that it has to do with a human subject, capable of intelligence and liberty. . . ."[18] Again, it is not clear what kinds of interventions or procedures would violate liberty in this sense, but it is notable that the problem of reductionism refers to a human capacity that is threatened either by being overridden or by being eliminated—the sense is unclear—by potential (although perhaps highly unlikely) uses of genetic technology.

Of course, both the papal declarations and the CBJC report represent a conservative position that many Catholic theologians do not accept. However, less conservative Catholic theologians reject genetic essentialism on similar grounds and draw similar conclusions regarding gene therapy. Considering whether genetic engineering alters human nature, Jean Porter argues that the characteristically human mode of life involves the subordination of biological processes to "the ongoing process of the rational formation and execution of purposes that is characteristic of human action."[19] No genetic intervention, then, can alter human nature unless it destroys the capacity for purposive action, and it is unclear how genetic engineering could accomplish such a result. Porter also concludes that even germ-line gene therapy is unlikely to affect human life as much as technological and cultural change do; the latter, presumably, more directly engage our purposive capacities.

For these Catholic commentators, then, humanity is defined in terms of a natural order, whether as a union of body and soul or a subordination of biological to purposive functions. Human beings exist in clear distinction from other forms of life, marked off by their charac teristic capacities. These definitions do not entail a rejection of genetic science: They are fully compatible with a recognition of the genetic basis of human traits (indeed, the ethical analysis in the papal declarations depends on the belief that genetic interventions may modify complex traits) and of the genetic kinship of all life forms. However, they do deny DNA a privileged role in characterizing human nature and personal identity; the genome is neither the essence of the human nor the locus of the dignity of the latter. Rather, that essence and that dignity are constituted by the ordering of body and soul or by the subordination of biological to purposive capacities. It follows that genetic interventions are problematic only insofar as they threaten to distort or obliterate this natural ordering that defines human nature.

This perspective also has implications for the distinction between therapy and enhancement in the context of genetic interventions, in effect subordinating (while retaining) this distinction to a more fundamental issue regarding the primacy of normal human functioning. The CBJC report defines health with reference to the contribution of "functional, goal-directed psychophysical systems," called "teleologies," to the good of the whole organism. Medical interventions are justifiable in cases of an "involuntary functional defect" in these teleologies, but are subject to a prima facie principle: that whenever possible, health should be promoted "through the normal channels of human *activity*, whether conscious or non-conscious."[20] In other words, medicine should intervene only when a functional defect renders the normal means to fulfillment unavailable or unsatisfactory. In the case of genetic interventions for purposes of enhancing human capacities, this amounts to a presumption in favor of "environmental" over "mechanical" interventions. The former involve "a mere *response* to *selected existing potential* of the child" and are "open-ended" in that they do not specify the exact characteristics or the degree to which the intervention will prove favorable. The latter, which include genetic interventions, involve "an *amendment* of existing potential" and "are something that *happens* to the child rather than something the child *does* in a certain environment."[21] This principle clearly draws a distinction between the natural and the artificial and expresses a valuation of the former over the latter. However, it is important not to confuse this distinction and preference with their counterparts under the concept of life itself. Natural and artificial correspond here (respectively) not to the living and the nonliving but to the exercise and circumvention of a natural ordering of human functions. The latter distinction is made possible by the concept of nature, not by that of life itself.

The distinctiveness of this account becomes clear when it is compared with more influential accounts that define health and disease and attempt to distinguish genetic therapy and enhancement in terms of a normal range of human functioning. According to many proponents of the latter type of account, interventions that bring capacities into the normal range are for that reason more easily justified than those that take capacities beyond the normal range or bring them to a higher level within the normal range. By contrast, what is normatively significant in the CBJC report is a functional ordering of nature, not a statistical range of the normal. The chief question here is when it is permissible or appropriate to interfere with or bypass the normal means of promoting human functioning. While the report does assign normative significance to the distinction between therapeutic and nontherapeutic uses of enhancement technologies, the crucial question in *both* cases is whether a defect or imperfection in functioning is important enough to justify overriding the presumption in favor of promoting functioning through the normal channels of human activity.[22]

Biotechnology and the Integrity of Life in Protestant and Ecumenical Statements

In contrast to these Catholic treatments of biotechnology, Protestant and ecumenical statements generally presuppose the concept of life itself. The following analysis focuses primarily on statements issued by the National Council of Churches (hereafter NCC), the World Council of Churches (hereafter WCC), and the United Methodist Church (hereafter UMC). These statements are the most comprehensive Protestant and ecumenical statements. In them, the Christian doctrine of creation is consistently explicated in terms of life, not natural order: "God is Creator of all life. Life is precious; therefore we must speak in faith to the manipulation of life forms."[23] Christology also is understood in terms of life: "The theological task ahead is to make sense of the claim that Christ is the unity of all life in the light of the new knowledge."[24] The new knowledge, of course, is genetic knowledge; because of the fundamental role of DNA in the concept of life itself, "[g]enetic science . . . explores the essence of life" and "develops means to alter the nature of life itself."[25] As with the Catholic statements, genetic science and technology raise for these Protestant and ecumenical statements troubling questions regarding human dignity and reductionism. However, while these concerns may appear to be the same, they sharply differ depending on whether they are determined by the concept of nature or that of life itself. In the Protestant and ecumenical statements, the problems regarding dignity and reductionism follow not from the possible eradication, distortion, or overriding of essentially human characteristics, but rather from certain implications of DNA as the essence of life. These implications are twofold. First, if DNA is the essence of human life, then the very act of intervening into it is problematic on two grounds: Interventions threaten a reduction of human life to mechanistic terms, and they threaten the very humanness of the human. Second, if DNA is the essence of human life, then the interconnectedness of all life through DNA threatens the uniqueness and moral status of human beings.

Because these Protestant and ecumenical statements understand creation in terms of life itself, the locus of the sacred shifts: It is no longer the ordering of living things but life itself that is sacred. However, if life itself, and not its order, is sacred, and DNA is the essence of life, the stage is set for a tension between the sacredness of life and its susceptibility to explanation in physical and chemical terms—a susceptibility that guarantees also its inherent manipulability.

> Life is holy because God is holy. This faith stance does not discount the scientists' assessment of life on a physico-chemical basis. Rather, it affirms the geneticist who also strives for the enhancement of life. And yet we must maintain the awareness that *life* is always the central issue when we speak of genetic engineering and recombinant-DNA technology. Such technology is never just the joining of "mere bits of matter."[26]

The danger is that life will be treated in thoroughly mechanistic terms, imperiling the appropriate awareness of the sacredness of life. The statement nevertheless endorses the mechanistic view insofar as it is in the service of enhancing life. However, the technology involved in enhancing life seems to be, crudely, "just the joining of 'mere bits of matter.' " What does it mean, then, in the exercise of this technology, to "maintain the awareness that *life* is always the central issue"? The tension between the concern to shield something of the sacredness of life from the mechanistic implications of genetic science and technology on the one hand, and from the threats genetic interventions pose to the human subject and human nature on the other hand, shouts louder than the confident affirmation of their compatibility, as the following considerations make clear.

Because DNA is both the essence of living things and capable of being treated in thoroughly mechanistic terms, genetic interventions involve a reductionism that threatens human dignity. "[I]f practiced directly and deliberately on human beings, genetic engineering converts the human subject into a composite object of interchangeable elements."[27] Of course, no major Protestant or ecumenical body argues from this reductionism to a prohibition of, or even a presumption against, genetic interventions; the potential the latter offer for the "enhancement of life," however that is to be defined (usually in a way that gives priority to the treatment of diseases), overrules the threat posed to human dignity by reductionism. However, reductionism is still a wrong or a harm done to the sacredness or dignity of human life; as such it would seem inevitably to leave a moral trace in every genetic intervention, however secure the ultimate justifiability of the latter.

The essential role of DNA in defining the human ensures that genetic interventions change human nature. Again, these ecclesial statements stop far short of prohibiting such interventions on these grounds, but at some point the threat to the humanness of the human becomes morally decisive. Often, this point is reached somewhere along the spectrum of germ-line interventions.

> Many ethical and religious traditions endorse some human freedom to modify or transcend nature. But for us to change *substantially* the germ-line DNA is to directly alter the genetic foundations of the human. In what ways do we, by manipulating our genes in other than simple ways, change ourselves to something less than human?[28]

Clearly, we have come a long way from the description of the genome as "simply one highly influential part of our bodies." Because DNA, and not an order of functions or capacities, most essentially characterizes the human, any alteration of DNA changes human nature. Unable to specify capacities whose loss or distortion would destroy human nature, and unwilling to prohibit germ-line interventions altogether, the *degree* of intervention becomes the morally decisive, if vague, criterion of what is morally acceptable and unacceptable.[29]

In short, for these Protestant and ecumenical bodies, genetic intervention itself—not the potential threat to the order of nature that might follow from a genetic intervention—is charged with moral significance. The significance follows from the fact that that which constitutes the essence of the human is susceptible to manipulation. Of course, the significance accorded to genetic interventions does not amount to a prohibition of, or even a presumption against, those interventions.

However, we have seen that the wrong or harm done to the human subject or to human nature as such by genetic interventions remains a factor, and at some point a decisive factor, in the ethical evaluation of the latter.

The reader will have noticed a slippage from the sacredness of life itself to the sacredness, or at least the dignity, of human life. This slippage occurs somewhat frequently, if unintentionally, in Protestant and ecumenical statements, and raises a question: If the knowledge of DNA forces on us the acknowledgment of the unity and interconnectedness of all life, on what grounds does one single out human dignity for special consideration? Are the concerns regarding reductionism and altering human nature relevant to all living things? These questions lead us to a problem that characterizes several of these ecclesial statements, but is especially apparent in a 1986 policy statement of the NCC. The immediate issue is the differing treatment given in the statement to animals on the one hand and "grains, vegetables and fruits" on the other hand. While acknowledging the fact that various techniques that accelerate processes of animal breeding have increased the food supply of "carnivorous humans,"[30] the statement goes on to register, although it does not endorse, various concerns with biotechnology as applied to animals. These concerns refer to shortcuts that violate "nature as given" in evolutionary processes and to "species integrity" and "the natural order of organisms" that is violated by crossing species barriers.[31]

It is worth pausing to sort out the range of concerns expressed here, which the statement appears to confuse. The concern to respect the givenness of nature renders intervention itself problematic (although it is not clear why genetic breeding at the molecular level, but not traditional methods of animal breeding, violates nature as given). This echoes the concern over altering human nature and would seem to extend the moral significance of intervention beyond humans to animals (although it is not clear on what grounds animals-as-they-are enjoy the same status, in this respect, as humanity-as-it-is enjoys). By contrast, the concerns regarding species integrity and the natural order of organisms are concerns of a different kind: They seem to follow not from the concept of life itself but from that of nature as an ordered system (although it is unclear whether certain kinds of hybrids, a certain degree of hybridization, or any hybridization at all violates the species integrity or natural order of animal life).

In any case, animals appear to have moral standing along with humans.[32] But when the statement turns to plants, the nature of moral concern shifts in a way that makes it clear that moral standing is ascribed not to nature as a whole but only to part of it. Genetic enhancement of grains, vegetables, and fruits "seem[s] to be of unambiguous value to humanity."[33] Rather than concerns for the integrity of natural processes or of species, the concerns here involve consequences (will genetic engineering reduce the variety of species to the extent that the food supply is rendered vulnerable to catastrophic diseases?) and economic justice (will concentrated ownership of patented plant products constitute an injustice against poor farmers?).

A similar distribution of value, along with a similar confusion between life itself and nature as an ordered system, can be found in the UMC statement. In assessing the relative merits of genetically enhanced bovine growth hormone and rotational grazing as alternative methods of increasing milk production, the statement proposes a criterion for deciding such issues: "Research stewardship requires that we be hesitant to make radical changes in the genetic structure of creation, especially when less intrusive and equally effective methods are available."[34] The statement expresses a preference, which apparently does not outweigh effectiveness but would presumably become decisive when two alternatives are equally effective, not to intervene into the genetic structures of organisms. Once again, intervention itself, the violation of the genetic structure of life as given in evolutionary processes—not the violation of a natural order—is the focus of moral concern. But why this preference for nongenetic interventions? Earlier, the statement affirms the importance of considering genetic science and technology "in accordance with our finite understanding of God's purposes for creation" and lists among these purposes "the integrity and ecological balance of creation."[35] In the present context, there is no reference to considerations of ecological balance, nor are any consequentialist reasons given for the preference not to intervene into genetic structures. It seems likely, then, that the preference for nongenetic interventions follows from the affirmation of the integrity of creation. Given the emphasis on DNA as the essence of life in the statement, it is not surprising that the genome turns out to be the site of this integrity.

But to what living things does this integrity apply? Once again, while terms like "integrity of creation" and "the genetic structure of creation" would lead us to conclude that the reference is to the living world as a whole, this is not the case. Near the end of the statement, note is taken of a concern "that genetic engineering will be used to help accommodate nature to the destructive habits of humans," for example by engineering wildlife capable of living in closer proximity to humans or in habitats destroyed by humans. The question is how far such engineering should go.

> While one or two gene transfers do not threaten the "pigness" of a pig, at some point a pig that contains enough genes from one or two other mammals including humans would cease to be a pig. . . . How many foreign genes should we permit to be transferred into organisms? How many human genes should we permit to be transferred into non-human organisms?[36]

Here the concern that genetic alterations, if substantial enough, change the nature of a living thing seems to extend beyond humans to take in animals as well, with the implication that a certain degree of intervention would be impermissible. The object of concern, however, is no longer the integrity of the genetic structure itself, but species integrity. And significantly, this concern over altering nature is never mentioned in the report's lengthy discussion of plants. Once again, the concerns raised by genetic interventions in plants are largely restricted to consequences and matters of economic justice.

These Protestant and ecumenical statements, then, exhibit a complex architecture. At one level there is a life-centered perspective rooted in the genetic interrelatedness, by virtue of DNA, of all organic beings that would lead one to believe that statements about the integrity of nature and its implications would apply to all life. "The intimate genetic relation of human beings to all other living matter, as well as the chemical relation to all matter as such, means that humans are a part of their own environment, even while transcending it."[37] If pursued consistently, this perspective would understand the sacredness of life in terms of respect for the genetic integrity of evolutionary processes. Concerns over reductionism and altering nature, as well as the tension between the sacredness or integrity of life on the one hand and the nature of DNA as a dynamic mechanism of interchangeable parts on the other hand, would apply across the entire spectrum of living beings, not just to humans and animals. These concerns would not necessarily entail the impermissibility of, or even a presumption against, all genetic interventions, but the reductionism involved in all such interventions would leave a moral trace, and at some point intervention would alter the givenness of nature to a degree that would be morally decisive against the intervention. However, while this perspective is consistent, it is ultimately incoherent, or at least the argument that would save it from incoherence has not been made. If DNA is the essence of life and is also inherently manipulable—if it is an exaggeration but not an absurdity for molecular biologists to claim that they are merely doing intentionally and purposefully what nature does blindly when they alter genetic structures—it is difficult to understand what it could mean to respect life in its evolutionary givenness, unless it is human agency itself, not the seemingly infinite alterability of these "mere bits of matter," that violates nature. In other words, if molecular biology is correct, there is no givenness of nature unless it is simply whatever has resulted so far from the infinite interchangeability of bits of matter; if human interventions are morally suspect, it must be because human agency, with its intentionality and its purposes, is suspect, not because such interventions alter nature. While it is not self-evidently absurd to argue that the givenness of nature even so understood has normative force and that intentional or purposive human actions must be defended in light of that force, no such argument appears in these ecclesial statements.

At another level the statements reveal an adherence to nature as an ordered system. This adherence is reflected in the hierarchy that places humans and animals, who alone are accorded intrinsic worth, over other living things, whose sole value is instrumental. "While holding to the primacy in value of all human life, we must respect animals for their own worth and do what is possible to preserve the earth's whole biosphere."[38] Although preservation could in this context indicate intrinsic value, the statements give few evidences of this. Rather, a line is drawn between humans and animals on one side, as those to whom the integrity of nature applies, and the rest of the living world on the other side, open for any form of genetic manipulation that respects social justice and passes consequentialist tests. Moreover, the integrity at stake here is not that of the givenness of evolutionary processes, but the purity of species. Here, however, the adherence to nature as an ordered system is incomplete: Species integrity is lost not when identifiable characteristic features that mark that species are eliminated or distorted, but when a sufficient amount of foreign DNA is transferred.[39] The genetic essentialism characteristic of the concept of life itself remains even when the order of nature is at stake. But once again, the infinite interchangeability of DNA, with or without human agency, renders the notion of species purity incoherent. Either the speed and/or the intentionality and purposiveness with which humans create hybrids is suspect, or hybridization crosses the moral barrier when it eliminates or distorts certain features regarded as fundamentally characteristic of the species—not when it merely transfers a certain amount of DNA.

Beyond Integrity: Re-Situating the Tension

If the claims regarding nature or life expressed in the ecclesial statements reviewed here adequately reflect the theology of the traditions or communities that produced the statements (a contestable assumption best left for theologians or other authorities who speak for those traditions or communities to debate), then we may expect that genuine conflicts between religion and biotechnology *on grounds of the integrity of nature or life* will be rare, at least in the case of these traditions and communities. (Of course, genuine conflicts may arise on other grounds, false conflicts may arise due to misunderstandings of a religious tradition by its adherents, and communities and traditions other than these may become involved in disputes with biotechnological practices or policies.) In the case of Roman Catholicism, such conflicts would apparently occur only with regard to interventions that are now hypothetical and implausible given present knowledge and technology. The case of Protestant and ecumenical bodies is more complex inasmuch as for them all interventions in humans and at least some interventions in animals pose threats, at least in principle, to the integrity of life. However, the statements stop short of a prohibition or even a presumption, on these grounds, against any interventions currently foreseeable.[40] It is possible that conflicts could arise over currently practiced genetic interventions with animals, but because references to animals in this connection are mostly expressions of ethical concern rather than articulations of principle, it is unclear where, or whether, lines could be drawn on the basis of these statements. It is true that the vague but constant threat that biotechnology poses to the integrity of life makes the stance of these Protestant and ecumenical communities toward biotechnology unstable, but the strong and enduring commitment of these traditions to healing, feeding, and generally meeting human needs almost guarantees that genuine conflicts over alleged violations of the integrity of life will be few and of short duration as long as biotechnological interventions are perceived as being effective in meeting human needs.

A different and more difficult question is whether the concerns over the integrity of nature or life expressed in these statements are the most adequate way for Christians to address what is at stake for them in biotechnology. The Roman Catholic strategy, at least as reflected in its official statements, has been to inscribe genetic knowledge and technology into an older understanding of natural order. While this strategy avoids the often-exaggerated claims for genetics as a master knowledge, it can also be accused of not taking seriously enough the challenges that the knowledges and practices connected with evolutionary and molecular biology have posed to "nature." By limiting the role the knowledges and practices that constitute biotechnology play in our interpretations of living things, including ourselves, these Catholic responses paradoxically diminish the opportunity for an effective challenge to the hegemony of these knowledges and practices over our lives. Only when we give biotechnology its due by acknowledging the place that it has come to play in our interpretations and practices can we begin to grapple with the question of what role it should play in those interpretations and practices.

The Protestant/ecumenical approach might seem more adequate from this perspective, but this appearance is misleading for two reasons. First, the engagement of theology with genetic science and technology often never occurs, and when it does it is either superficial or one-sided. That is, theological claims are either (1) juxtaposed to claims regarding genetic science and technology without any effort to reconcile the two discourses, as in many discussions of human dignity; (2) selectively and without analysis used to restate aspects of genetic science or technology in religious language, as in the numerous uses of the term *imago Dei*; or (3) required to undergo reinterpretation (seldom actually carried out) to make them compatible with genetic science and technology, as in the repeated reminders in the UMC statement of the power of developments in genetic science to "compel our reevaluation of accepted theological/ethical issues including determinism vs. free will, the nature of sin, just distribution of resources, the status of human beings in relation to other forms of life, and the meaning of personhood."[41] Second, the development of biotechnology itself renders the concept of life itself questionable. Ironically, DNA has proven to be just as effective in undermining the very notion of life itself as it was indispensable to conceptualizing the latter. As Franklin notes, "insofar as the biogenetic definition of life relies on an informational model, of DNA as a message or code, the distinction between life and nonlife is readily challenged by complex informational systems that are to a degree self-regulating and that have the capacity both to replicate themselves and to evolve."[42] In Donna Haraway's terms, life in the era of molecular biology "is constituted and connected by recursive, repeating streams of information."[43] If the concept of life itself is founded on the distinction between the natural (understood in terms of features such as growth, evolution, and self-reproduction) and the artificial, then biotechnology has destroyed the concept of life itself. In addition to the informational systems to which Franklin alludes, the distinction is also obliterated by the inability to distinguish meaningfully between knowing living things in molecular terms and remaking them, or (as noted above) between the remaking the scientist does in her laboratory and the remaking that occurs apart from human agency.

Does this leave any room at all for conceptions of the integrity of nature or life? Commenting on some of the trends just mentioned, Paul Rabinow coins the suggestive term "biosociality" to indicate the modeling (and remaking) of nature according to culture in contrast to sociobiology, which tried to model (and remake?) culture according to nature.[44] Rabinow's wide-ranging essay points out how biotechnology knows and remakes nature in terms of cultural practices and norms, breaking down the distinction between culture and nature. Just as, in Rabinow's analysis, biotechnology has redescribed and remade the tomato in accordance with consumer tastes and biopolitical norms such as nutrition, so will likely go much (most? all?) of the rest of what we call nature. If nature is being redescribed and remade in accordance with human aims, desires, and norms, a Christian ethic of biotechnology has two important tasks in addition to concerns about risks, harms, and distributive justice. One task is to carry out, where appropriate, the critique of those aims, desires, and norms and to resist and appropriate (and prioritize) biotechnological developments in ways that further the self- and other-regarding commitments of Christian ethics. The other task is to affirm, against the incremental utopianism of much of the biotechnology industry, the intractable otherness of nature that on this side of the resurrection resists the totalizing union with human aims, desires, and norms. While there is little reason to fear that a biotechnological utopia will be any more successful at supplanting Christian eschatology than were any other utopias of recent centuries—that eschatology has perhaps more to fear from the rejection of all efforts to improve human life, which in their overemphasis on the absence of the "not yet" deny the equally important presence of the "already"—there is much to fear from a refusal to acknowledge the extent to which nature, even as we construct it, exceeds our knowledge and control, and to grant this intractable otherness of nature its place in our deliberations.

NOTES

1. Francis Crick, co-discoverer of the DNA molecule, correlates belief in vitalism with religious, and especially Roman Catholic, belief. See Francis Crick, *Of Molecules and Men* (Seattle: University of Washington Press, 1966).

2. See World Council of Churches, *Biotechnology: Its Challenges to the Churches and the World* (Geneva: World Council of Churches, 1989).

3. Use of the language of the sacred in connection with DNA is, in one form or another, fairly widespread in both popular culture and among scientists, as Dorothy Nelkin and Susan Lindee document. See Dorothy Nelkin and Susan Lindee, *The DNA Mystique:The Gene as Cultural Icon* (New York: W. H. Freeman, 1995).

4. By a genuine conflict between religion and biotechnology, I mean one that involves important religious convictions, whether or not such a conflict is ever made explicit or public, and whether or not the recognized leaders or a significant number of the members of a community that in principle adheres to that conviction identify it as a conflict.

5. I identify some of these problems in some recent discussions of the body in biomedical ethics. See Gerald P. McKenny, "The Integrity of the Body: Critical Remarks on a Persistent Theme in Bioethics," in *Persons and Their Bodies: Rights, Responsibilities, Relationships*, ed. Thomas Bole and Mark J. Cherry (Dordrecht: Kluwer Academic Publishers, 1999), pp. 353–61.

6. I have deliberately stated these possible kinds of order in a way that includes both "physicalist" versions of natural law and "personalist" restatements of the latter in contemporary Roman Catholic theology and official teaching. For example, in opposition to views that describe the body as extrinsic to the person, Pope John Paul II affirms the place of the body in the unity of the person as a whole. From this perspective, he attempts to restate moral principles drawn from physicalist theories of natural order in personalist terms. See Pope John Paul II, *Veritatis Splendor*, #48–50.

7. Leon R. Kass, *Toward a More Natural Science: Biology and Human Affairs* (New York: Free Press, 1985).

8. The following description is influenced by Michel Foucault, *The Order of Things: An Archaeology of the Human Sciences* (New York: Random House, 1970 [1966]); Sarah Franklin, "Life," in *Encyclopedia of Bioethics* (New York: Macmillan, 1995), pp. 1345–52; and Donna J. Haraway, *Modest_Witness@ Second_Millenium.FemaleMan_Meets_OncoMouse: Feminism and Technoscience* (New York: Routledge, 1997). Its particular form, emphases, and details, however, follow from my reading of the ecclesial statements themselves, along with other texts that exhibit similar features.

9. Franklin, "Life," p. 1347.

10. Hans Jonas, *The Phenomenon of Life: Toward a Philosophical Biology* (New York: Harper and Row, 1966).

11. Franklin, "Life," p. 1347.

12. Hans Jonas argued forcefully against the sufficiency of mechanistic explanations of life on similar grounds. See Jonas, *The Phenomenon of Life.*

13. Franklin, "Life," p. 1346. See Richard Dawkins, *The Selfish Gene*, new ed. (New York: Oxford University Press, 1989), pp. 1–45.

14. While the conviction of the sacredness of DNA is often portrayed as a mere remainder of a prescientific era or a nostalgic return to the archaic—as a failure to embrace the mechanistic reductionism demanded by a consistently scientific approach—we are left, I believe, with the conclusion that sacred DNA, no less than Dawkins' gene/soul, is the product of a peculiarly modern concept of life that is inevitably bound up with categories and concepts of long-standing importance in the West.

15. Catholic Bishops' Joint Committee on Bioethical Issues, *Genetic Intervention on Human Subjects: The Report of a Working Party* (London: Linacre Centre, 1995), p. 32. While this report does not claim to represent official Catholic teaching on the matters it investigates, its episcopal connection gives it some authority.

16. Pope John Paul II, "Biological Research and Human Dignity," *Origins* 12 (1982): 342–43; Pope John Paul II, "The Ethics of Genetic Manipulation," *Origins* 13 (1983): 385–89.

17. Pope John Paul II, "The Ethics of Genetic Manipulation," pp. 387–88.

18. Pope John Paul II, "The Ethics of Genetic Manipulation," p. 388.

19. Jean Porter, "What Is Morally Distinctive about Genetic Engineering?" *Human Gene Therapy* 1 (1990): 419–24, at 422.

20. Catholic Bishops Joint Committee on Bioethical Issues, *Genetic Intervention on Human Subjects*, p. 22.

21. Catholic Bishops Joint Committee on Bioethical Issues, *Genetic Interventions on Human Subjects*, pp. 39–40.

22. While the distinction between normal activity and mechanical intervention is not without problems, it is frequently confused with a very different distinction between the natural and the artificial. This confusion can lead to serious misunderstandings. For example, a prominent genetic ethicist argued at the 1997 Gene Therapy Policy Conference sponsored by the National Institutes of Health that it is illegitimate for people to claim that pharmacological interventions are artificial while, say, meditation or psychotherapy is natural. There is some truth in this if one identifies nature with the physical or biochemical, to which meditation or psychotherapy might be contrasted (provided the contrast is not drawn too sharply). However, the Bishops Joint Committee obviously does not make this identification. For members of the committee, conscious and unconscious activity are as natural to human beings as is their biochemistry.

23. Frank Harron, ed., *Genetic Engineering: Social and Ethical Consequences* (New York: Pilgrim Press, 1984), p. 21. This book is the report of a committee convened by the National Council of Churches.

24. World Council of Churches, *Manipulating Life* (Geneva: World Council of Churches, 1982), p. 2.

25. United Methodist Church, "United Methodist Church Genetic Science Task Force Report to the 1992 General Conference," *Church and Society* 18 (1992): 113–23, at 115–16.

26. Harron, *Genetic Engineering*, p. 21.

27. World Council of Churches, *Manipulating Life*, p. 8.

28. World Council of Churches, *Manipulating Life*, p. 8.

29. A small minority of Protestants, mostly Europeans, go even further, arguing that any germ-line intervention would violate the genetic integrity of the human or offend against the notion that humanity as it is, is created in the image of God. See K. von Kooten Niekerk, "Die Diskussion in Skandinavien," in *Biotechnologie und Evangelische Ethik*, ed. Johann Hueber and Hartwig von Schubert (Frankfurt: Campus Verlag, 1992), pp. 289–378, at 344-46.

30. Technically, human beings, which as a species eat vegetables and grains as well as meat, are omnivores rather than carnivores.

31. National Council of the Churches of Christ in the U.S.A., *Genetic Science for Human Benefit* (New York: National Council of the Churches of Christ in the U.S.A., 1986), p. 7.

32. This does not mean that the only concern here is animal-regarding; the statement goes on to note an additional human-regarding concern "that genetic and reproductive manipulation of animals presages the same with human beings" due to their common mammalian bodies.

33. National Council of the Churches of Christ in the U.S.A., *Genetic Science for Human Benefit*, p. 8.

34. United Methodist Church, "Genetic Science Task Force Report," p. 117.

35. United Methodist Church, "Genetic Science Task Force Report," p. 115.

36. United Methodist Church, "Genetic Science Task Force Report," p. 121.

37. National Council of the Churches of Christ in the U.S.A., *Genetic Science for Human Benefit*, p. 13.

38. National Council of the Churches of Christ in the U.S.A., *Genetic Science for Human Benefit*, p. 13.

39. A careful reader of these statements might object that quantity of DNA serves not as a criterion here but rather as a proxy for functions or characteristics that in fact define species but are difficult to determine with precision. In an appendix to *Manipulating Life*, the WCC seems to have precisely this in mind, arguing that it is not the quantity of transferred DNA that is morally troubling about human-animal hybrids but the deliberate production of a human being who lacks certain features, impossible to delimit with precision, that normal human beings possess (World Council of Churches,

Manipulating Life, pp. 28–30). This of course raises numerous questions, but at this point I am interested only in the possibility that the WCC regards the essence of human life in terms of a real but unspecifiable class of phenotypical characteristics rather than in terms of a genome. If so, and aside from other problems, it is still unclear exactly how quantity of DNA stands as a proxy for these real but unspecifiable characteristics, and why the statement fails to explain the role of quantity of DNA as proxy when it refers (p. 8) to the degree of intervention as a possible wrong-making feature of some forms of human germ-line gene therapy.

40. The preference for nongenetic interventions as advocated in the UMC statement might appear to be an exception to this conclusion, but a preference for one thing does not amount to a presumption against an alternative. I can prefer, for the reasons the UMC statement mentions, to accomplish a desired result by traditional breeding rather than gene transfer when the costs and benefits of each procedure are roughly equal, without claiming that gene transfers are *prima facie* wrong.

41. See, respectively, National Council of the Churches of Christ in the U.S.A., *Human Life and the New Genetics* (New York: National Council of the Churches of Christ in the U.S.A., 1980), p. 45; United Methodist Church, "Genetic Science Task Force Report," p. 115.

42. Franklin, "Life," p. 1348.

43. Haraway, *Modest_Witness@Second_Millenium*, p. 134.

44. Paul Rabinow, "Artificiality and Enlightenment: From Sociobiology to Biosociality," in *Incorporations*, ed. Jonathan Crary and Sanford Kwinter (New York: Zone, 1992), pp. 234–52.

ELLIOT N. DORFF

Jewish Views on Technology in Health Care[1]

Judaism, a religion tracing its roots to Abraham close to 4,000 years ago and continuing through the Bible and rabbinic interpretations to our own day, has sought since its inception to use the world productively while yet preserving it, both seen as God's commands. This essay first describes the theological foundations for Judaism's activist, and yet respectful, stance toward the world and toward life and health. It then focuses on how this stance is articulated in issues at the beginning of life, both in current practice and in research. Issues at the end of life, including artificial nutrition and hydration, life-support machines like ventilators, and organ transplantation, are no less interesting, but the newest issues in biotechnology—like cloning and stem cell research—argue for focusing on the beginning of life within the limitations of space of this chapter.[2]

Jewish Theological and Moral Moorings

On Methodology
The Jewish tradition uses both theology and law to discern what God wants of us. No legal theory that ignores the theological convictions of Judaism is adequate to the task, for such theories lead to blind legalism without a sense of the law's context or purpose. Conversely, no theology that ignores Jewish law can speak authoritatively for the Jewish tradition, for Judaism places great trust in law as a means to discriminate moral differences in similar cases, thus giving us moral guidance.

On Technology Generally
Adam and Eve are told in the Garden of Eden "to work it and to preserve it" (Genesis 2:15). Judaism has ever since tried to strike a *balance* between using the world for human purposes while still safeguarding and

sustaining it. We are not supposed to desist from changing the world altogether: "Six days shall you do your work" is as much a commandment as "and on the seventh day you shall rest [literally, desist]" (Exodus 23:12).

In changing the world to accomplish our ends, though, we must take care to preserve the environment, whether we are practicing medicine, farming, travelling, or doing anything else. This balance is demanded because, in the end, we do not own the world; God does.[3] We are but tenants in God's world, with a lease on life and on the world.

During the duration of that lease, we may and should act as God's agents to improve it. God, in fact, intended that we function in that way. This is probably most starkly stated in a rabbinic comment about, of all things, circumcision. If God wanted all Jewish boys circumcised, the rabbis ask, why did He not create them that way? The answer, according to the rabbis, is that God deliberately created the world in need of fixing so that human beings would have a divinely ordained task in life, thus giving human life purpose and meaning.[4] We are, then, not only permitted, but mandated to find ways to bend God's world to God's purposes and ours—as long, again, as we preserve God's world in the process.

Thus technology, in and of itself, is not good or bad: it depends upon how we use it. If we employ it to assist us in bending the world to morally good ends while yet preserving the world, our use of technology is theologically approved and morally good. If, on the other hand, we disregard our duty to preserve the world when using technological tools, we are engaged in a theologically and morally bad act.

On Health Care

When we turn now specifically to biotechnology and to the branch of it relating to health care, three underlying principles emerge from Jewish sources.[5]

God's ownership of our bodies.   Since God owns everything in the world, our bodies are not ours. Rather, God loans our bodies to us for the duration of our lives, and they are returned to God when we die.

The immediate implication of this principle is that neither men nor women have the right to use their bodies as they will. Since God created our bodies and owns them, God can and does assert the right to govern the care and use of our bodies. Thus Jewish law requires us to safeguard our health and life,[6] and, conversely, to avoid danger and injury.[7] So, for example, Conservative, Reform, and some Orthodox authorities have prohibited smoking as an unacceptable risk to our God-owned bodies.[8] Ultimately, human beings do not, according to Judaism, have the right to dispose of their bodies at will (i.e., commit suicide), for that would be a total obliteration of that which does not belong to them but rather belongs to God.[9]

The body's status and function.   The second major principle underlying Jewish medical ethics is that the body is morally neutral and potentially good. For Judaism the body is as much the creation of God as the mind, the will, the emotions, and the spirit are. Its energies, like those of our other faculties, are morally neutral, but they can and should be used for divine purposes as defined by Jewish law and tradition. Within that structure, the body's pleasures are God-given and are not to be shunned, for that would be an act of ingratitude toward our Creator.[10] The body, in other words, can and should give us pleasure to the extent that that fits within its overriding purpose of enabling us to live a life of holiness.

The Jewish mode for attaining holiness is to use all of our faculties, including our bodily energies, to perform God's commandments. Maimonides (1135–1204) states this well:

> He who regulates his life in accordance with the laws of medicine with the sole motive of maintaining a sound and vigorous physique and begetting children to do his work and labor for his benefit is not following the right course. A man should aim to maintain physical health and vigor in order that his soul may be upright, in a condition to know God. . . . Whoever throughout his life follows this course will be continually serving God, even while engaged in business and even during cohabitation, because his purpose in all that he does will be to satisfy his needs so as to have a sound body with which to serve God. Even when he sleeps and seeks repose to calm his mind and rest his body so as not to fall sick and be incapacitated from serving God, his sleep is service of the Almighty.[11]

The medical and technological implications of this are clear. Jews have the obligation to maintain health not only to care for God's property, but also so that they can accomplish their purpose in life, that is, to live a life of holiness. Moreover, since pain is not perceived as a method of attaining holiness but is rather an impediment to acting according to God's law, it is our duty to relieve it. Thus perhaps the most pervasive corollary of Judaism's insistence on the divine source of our bodies is its positive attitude toward the body and medicine.

The role of medicine.
The role of medicine.   God's ownership of our bodies is also behind our obligation to help other people escape sickness, injury, and death.[12] God is our ultimate healer, as the Bible asserts in many places,[13] but God both authorizes us and commands us to aid in that process.[14] In fact, the duty of saving a life (*pikkuah nefesh*) takes precedence over all but three of the commandments in the Torah.[15]

The Talmud reflects some ambivalence about the level of expertise of physicians of its time (most explicitly in comments like "The best of physicians deserve to go to Hell!"), and some later Jewish authorities were particularly wary of physicians' abilities to practice internal medicine (in contrast to surgery and healing external wounds and diseases). In the end, though, the Talmud prohibits Jews from living in a community in which there is no physician. Here this third principle wraps back into the first, for if we were not within easy reach of a doctor, we could not as effectively carry out our fiduciary obligation to God to take care of our bodies.[16]

Medical experts, in turn, have special obligations because of their expertise. Thus Rabbi Joseph Karo (1488–1575), the author of one of the most important Jewish codes, says this:

> The Torah gave permission to the physician to heal; moreover, this is a religious precept and is included in the category of saving life, and if the physician withholds his services, it is considered as shedding blood.[17]

The following rabbinic story indicates that the rabbis recognized the theological issue involved in medical care and in the use of technology generally, but it also indicates the clear assertion of the Jewish tradition that the use of technology to assist in good purposes like producing food and preserving health is legitimate and, in fact, obligatory:

> It once happened that Rabbi Ishmael and Rabbi Akiva were strolling in the streets of Jerusalem accompanied by another person. They were met by a sick person. He said to them, "My masters, tell me by what means I may be cured." They told him, "Do thus and so until you are cured." The sick man asked them, "And who afflicted me?" They replied, "The Holy One, blessed be He." The sick man responded, "You have entered into a matter which does not pertain to you. God has afflicted, and you seek to cure! Are you not transgressing His will?"

Rabbi Akiva and Rabbi Ishmael asked him, "What is your occupation?" The sick man answered, "I am a tiller of the soil, and here is the sickle in my hand." They asked him, "Who created the vineyard?" "The Holy One, blessed be He," he answered. Rabbi Akiva and Rabbi Ishmael said to him, "You enter into a matter which does not pertain to you! God created the vineyard, and you cut fruits from it."

He said to them, "Do you not see the sickle in my hand? If I did not plow, sow, fertilize, and weed, nothing would sprout."

Rabbi Akiva and Rabbi Ishmael said to him, "Foolish man!

. . . Just as if one does not weed, fertilize, and plow, the trees will not produce fruit, and if fruit is produced but is not watered or fertilized, it will not live but die, so with regard to the body. Drugs and medicaments are the fertilizer, and the physician is the tiller of the soil.[18]

The rabbis quite explicitly, then, understand God to depend upon us to aid in the process of healing. We are, in the talmudic phrase, God's partners in the ongoing act of creation.[19]

Underlying Principles Regarding Family, Sexuality, and Procreation[20]

Marriage and children are the epitome of blessing in the Jewish view. "It is not good for man to live alone," the Torah declares, and so one goal of marriage is companionship, sexual and otherwise.[21]

The second goal of marriage is procreation. Children figure prominently in the Bible's descriptions of life's chief goods,[22] and so God's blessings of the Patriarchs promise numerous children.[23] Procreation is not only a blessing; it is a commandment. Indeed, the very first commandment in the Bible is "Be fruitful and multiply" (Genesis 1:28). In rabbinic interpretation, for exegetical and probably economic reasons, it is the man who bears the responsibility to propagate, even though men obviously cannot do so without women. A man, then, fulfills the obligation to propagate when he fathers minimally two children, and since we are supposed to model ourselves after God, the ideal is to have both a boy and a girl, thus creating both male and female, just as God did (Genesis 1:27).[24] One should, though, have as many children as one can.

The family is important in Judaism not only because it is in that context that adults gain sexual fulfillment and the next generation is produced; it is also important because it is in the family that the tradition is passed on. Parents have a biblical obligation to teach the tradition to their children,[25] and even after schools were established in the first century, parents remained ultimately responsible for the education of their children.

Preventing Conception

Contraception

With the importance of marriage and children in mind, one can understand that traditional Judaism looked askance at interruptions in the process of conception and birth. Normally one was supposed to marry and have children. Birth control, sterilization, and abortion were, both physically and ideologically, counterproductive.

Until very recently, the use of birth control or even abortion for family planning purposes, so common in our day, was simply unknown to the tradition. Methods of birth control—either a cloth inserted in the vaginal cavity or a "cup of roots" taken orally—were unreliable, and abortion posed a major threat to the life of the woman. Moreover, if a couple wanted to have two or three children survive to adulthood, they had to produce six or seven. We must keep in mind this major distinction in context and purpose, then, when we examine and evaluate traditional Jewish sources on methods of preventing conception.

The rabbis state that the methods of contraception they had are permitted and even required under certain circumstances. Because the tradition understands the command to propagate to be the obligation of the male, male forms of contraception are generally forbidden. The specific conditions under which female contraception is permitted (and, in some cases, even required) depend upon one's interpretation of a second-century rabbinic ruling describing three classes of women who "use" contraceptives—namely, a minor (less than twelve years of age), a pregnant woman, and a nursing woman. The present tense of the verb is ambiguous in Hebrew, as it is in English. If it means that these women *must* use contraceptives to protect their life or health or that of their nursing infant, women in other circumstances then *may* use contraceptives. On the other hand, if these three categories of women *may* use contraceptives only to preserve life and health, then when that is not a factor, women *may not* use contraceptives.[26] In any case, because Judaism restricts the legitimacy of abortion to cases where the life or health of the mother is at stake, modern forms of contraception that prevent conception in the first place (e.g., the pill, the diaphragm) are preferred over those that abort the fertilized egg cell after the fact (e.g., RU486).

Sterilization

The same concerns govern the issue of sterilization, but there another issue arises, namely, the prohibition against a person mutilating his or her body in light of the fact that the body is really God's property. Although the procedures are rather new, there are a few rabbinic rulings available on the issues of vasectomies and tubal ligations. Both traditional and liberal respondents forbid male sterilization on the basis of the rabbinic interpretation and extension of Deuteronomy 23:2 ("No one whose testes are crushed . . . shall be admitted into the congregation of the Lord"),[27] or Leviticus 22:24 ("That which is mauled or crushed or torn or cut you shall not offer unto the Lord; nor shall you do this in your land").[28] They are more permissive about female sterilization, both because a woman does not come under those prohibitions and also because she is not legally obligated to procreate.[29]

All sources agree, however, that even male sterilization is permitted and perhaps even required if the man's life or health makes it necessary, as, for example, if he contracts testicular cancer. Moreover, even though I am not aware of any written opinion that would allow a vasectomy, I could imagine an argument consistent with Jewish law and principles that would permit a vasectomy when pregnancy would entail a severe risk to the man's wife. After all, that procedure is far easier and safer than tying a woman's tubes, and saving a person's life takes precedence over both the commandment to procreate and the prohibition of injuring oneself. Moreover, a vasectomy does not amount to castration or to crushing the testes, and so the biblical verses cited above are not directly violated by the operation. The question, though, would be whether pregnancy could be effectively prevented by other means that would not endanger the woman and would not even possibly violate the verses cited. If so, then such means would undoubtedly be preferable.

Most often, though, men contemplate vasectomies simply because they do not want to father any more children. In light of the strong bias of the Jewish tradition for having children, and in light of the major demographic crisis facing the Jewish community that I shall describe below, rabbis have not endorsed vasectomies for family planning purposes, seeing it as a violation of Jewish law and values and a threat to the continuity of the Jewish people.

Abortion

There is a clear bias for life within the Jewish tradition. Indeed, it is considered sacred. Consequently, although abortion is permitted in some circumstances and actually required in others, it is not viewed as a morally neutral matter of individual desire or an acceptable form of *post facto* birth control. Contrary to what many contemporary Jews think, Judaism restricts the legitimacy of abortion to a narrow range of cases; it does not permit abortion at will.

Judaism does not see all abortion as murder, as Catholicism does, because biblical and rabbinic sources understand the process of gestation developmentally. Thus Exodus 21:22-25 makes a clear distinction between an assailant who causes miscarriage of a fetus, when only monetary fines are imposed, as opposed to one who causes the death of the mother, when the rule is "life for life." According to the Talmud, within the first forty days after conception the zygote is "simply water." Another talmudic source distinguishes the first trimester from the rest of pregnancy.[30] After the first forty days or first trimester, the child is, according to the Talmud, "like the thigh of its mother."[31] It is not a theory of ensoulment that determines these marking points; it is rather the physical development of the fetus.

The effect of these demarcations is to make abortion during the early periods permitted for more reasons than during the rest of pregnancy.[32] Classifying the first forty days of gestation as "simply water," though, does not amount to a blanket permission to abort. Thus the RU486 pill, advertised as a "morning after pill" for those couples who simply do not want to have a baby, would be forbidden as a *post facto* contraceptive. On the other hand, if the woman's life or health would be threatened by pregnancy, then use of the RU486 pill would be preferable to a later-term abortion, both because it poses less risk for the woman and because the fetus is further from becoming a full human being.

During the second stage of pregnancy the fetus is like the thigh of its mother. Neither men nor women may amputate their thigh at will, for that would injure their body that belongs to God. Thus, abortion is generally prohibited in Jewish law, not as an act of murder (for the fetus becomes a human being only at birth), but as an act of self-injury. If a person's thigh had turned gangrenous, however, and if there were no way to save the life or health of the person except by amputating the leg, one would be required to undergo that operation in order to save one's life. Similarly, if the fetus threatens the mother's life or health, she *must* undergo an abortion. Finally, when pregnancy poses a risk to the woman greater than that of normal pregnancy but less than a clear and present danger to her life and health, then she may take the risk and carry the fetus to term, or she *may* avoid the risk by aborting the pregnancy. Thus, abortion is sometimes required in Jewish law and sometimes permitted, but it is generally forbidden.

The fetus does not attain the full rights and protections of a human being until birth, specifically when the forehead emerges or, if it is a breech birth, when most of the body emerges.[33] The mother, of course, has full human status. Consequently, if the fetus threatens the life or health of the mother, then it may and in some cases must be aborted, as the following Mishnah graphically stipulates: "If a woman has (life-threatening) difficulty in childbirth, one dismembers the embryo in her, limb by limb, because her life takes precedence over its life. Once its head (or its 'greater part') has emerged, it may not be touched, for we do not set aside one life for another."[34]

While all Jewish sources would permit and even require abortion in order to preserve the life or organs of the mother,[35] authorities differ widely on how much of a threat to a woman's health the fetus must pose to justify or require an abortion. Based on a responsum by Rabbi Israel Meir Mizrahi in the late seventeenth century, many modern authorities also permit an abortion to preserve the mother's mental health, and this has been variously construed in narrow or lenient terms in modern times.[36] To the extent that Jewish law makes special provision for an unusually young or old mother, an unmarried mother, the victim of a rape, or the participant in an adulterous or incestuous union, abortion is construed to preserve the mother's mental health.[37]

There is no justification in the traditional sources for aborting a fetus for reasons having to do with the health of the fetus; only the mother's health is a consideration. As a result, some rabbis object to performing an amniocentesis at all, even when the intent is to determine whether to abort a malformed fetus.[38] Others reason in precisely the opposite direction. They point out that the sources could not have contemplated abortions due to the condition of the fetus because nobody could know anything about that until very recently through technologies like amniocentesis and sonograms. Now that we have those tools, most rabbis justify using them to aid in the delivery of a healthy baby. Moreover, when those technologies reveal fetal abnormalities, many rabbis justify abortion on the basis of preserving the mother's mental health where it is clear that the mother is not able to cope with the prospect of bearing or raising such a child.[39]

Many Conservative and Reform rabbis, and even a few contemporary Orthodox rabbis, have handled the matter in a completely different way. Our new medical knowledge of the status of the fetus, they say, ought to establish the fetus' health as an independent consideration in determining when abortion is justified.[40]

In practice much of this discussion is moot, for Jews engage in abortion as if it were a matter of individual choice. That is a particularly problematic phenomenon for the contemporary Jewish community because Jews constitute only 0.2 percent of the world's population (while Christians make up a full 33 percent). To make matters worse, Jews are barely reproducing themselves in Israel and are falling far short of that in North America, where the Jewish reproductive rate is approximately 1.6 or 1.7 children per couple. Consequently, even those rabbis who are liberal in their interpretation of Jewish abortion law are also calling for Jews to marry and to have children so that the Jewish people and Judaism can survive.

Generating Conception

Artificial Insemination

Since Judaism prizes children so much, it is no wonder that rabbinic authorities have permitted unusual ways of having them for couples who cannot have them otherwise. Nevertheless there are objections, or at least precautions, connected to some of the procedures.

Rabbis have not objected to uniting a man's sperm with his wife's ovum artificially, whether through artificial insemination or through in vitro fertilization (IVF).[41] Because of Judaism's appreciation of medicine as an aid to God, there is no abhorrence of such means merely because they are artificial.

The matter becomes more complicated when the donor is not the husband. Some rabbis object to such procedures on grounds of adultery. For many, however, adultery takes place only when the penis of the man enters the vaginal cavity of the woman, and that is clearly not the case when insemination takes place artificially. Not only is the physical contact missing; the intent to have an illicit relationship is also absent.[42]

More commonly, the objection to donor insemination is based on the possibility of unintentional incest in the next generation—specifically, if the product of the artificial insemination later happens to fall in love with a person of the opposite sex who is the child the semen donor conceived with his wife. Since their biological father is the same man, these two people would be each other's biological half-brother or half-sister. That is problematic for some because it represents a violation of the Torah's laws against incest (Leviticus 18:9; 20:17). Even for those who would invoke the lack of intent to excuse the couple from those laws, there still remains a critical health concern—namely, the increased likelihood among consanguineous unions of genetic diseases transferring from one generation to the next.

This issue dissolves if the semen donor is known or if the donor would not likely be a marital partner for someone in the Jewish community. It was on the latter basis that a prominent Orthodox rabbi, Rabbi Moshe Feinstein, ruled that donor insemination would be permissible if the donor were not Jewish, for in his community intermarriage between Jews and non-Jews was rare. Those Orthodox Jews who use donor insemination therefore often require that the donor be a non-Jew.

The Conservative Movement's Committee on Jewish Law and Standards has approved my rabbinic ruling, according to which donor insemination is permissible if either the identity of the donor is known or, lacking that, that enough is known about him so that the child can avoid unintentional incest in his or her sexual partners (married or not) and so that the child can know as much as possible about his or her family traits, both medically and characterologically. In view, however, of the psychological problems that may ensue for the child, the donor, and/or the parents who raise the child (the "social parents"), all parties to the insemination should seek and receive appropriate counseling.[43]

Egg Donation

The considerations described above with regard to donor insemination apply as well to egg donation. If the identity of the egg donor remains confidential, the same problems arise with regard to possible unintentional incest in the next generation, and the same solutions by the various rabbinic authorities apply. Specifically, either the egg donor's identity should be shared with the couple who will raise the child and ultimately with the child him/herself, or the woman should be a non-Jew, or enough about the biological mother must be shared with the couple and child to enable the child to avoid such unintentional incest. The donor, in my view, also must share enough information about her talents and traits to help the child understand her/himself. Finally, psychological counseling is appropriate for all concerned both before the procedure and afterward.

Egg donation, though, raises some additional problems. Semen donors incur virtually no medical risks, but that is not true of egg donors. In order to procure as many eggs as possible during each attempt, the donor must be hyperovulated with drugs, and there is some evidence that repeated hyperovulation increases the risk of ovarian cancer.[44] This is especially troubling since the donor herself will not, by hypothesis, be gaining a child of her own but will rather be helping another couple have a child. For all that Jewish law prizes procreation, it values the life and health of those already born even more. Consequently, while healthy women may undergo the procedure to donate eggs once or twice, they may not do so much more than that, unless new studies allay the fear of increased cancer risk.

Normally, a child is defined as Jewish in traditional Jewish law if born to a Jewish woman. In cases of egg donation, some rabbis have maintained that it is the donor of the gametes who is the legal mother. Most, though, have ruled that even if the egg comes from some other woman, as it does in egg donation, it is the bearing mother whose religion determines whether the child is Jewish or not, and the Conservative Movement's Committee on Jewish Law and Standards has adopted that view.[45]

In Vitro Fertilization (IVF), Gamete Intrauterine Fallopian Transfer (GIFT), Zygote Intrauterine Fallopian Transfer (ZIFT), etc.

When a couple cannot conceive a fetus through sexual intercourse, even when assisted by timing their intercourse, by stimulating ovulation, or by surgery to correct a problem in either the man or the woman, and when the couple prefers to use their own gametes to those of donors, they may try any of a number of new techniques, some of which are listed in the title of this subsection. Since the Jewish tradition does not frown upon the use of artificial means to enable people to attain permissible ends, much less sanctified ones like having a child, the mechanical nature of these techniques is not an issue. On the contrary, the important thing to note in recent Jewish rulings is that infertile couples are *not obligated* to use these means to fulfill the man's duty to procreate, even though they *may*.[46]

If they use their own gametes in these procedures, no problems arise. If they use donor gametes, the same problems and solutions occur as described in the section above on artificial insemination.

When a woman is impregnated with more than three fetuses, either naturally or artificially, an abortion may be indicated in order to preserve both the life of the mother and the viability and health of the remaining fetuses. For the latter purpose, an abortion is permitted, and for the former, an abortion is required. When it can be determined through genetic testing that some of the fetuses have a greater chance to survive and to be healthy than others, then it is permissible selectively to abort those less likely to survive. This is the same criterion to be used for triage decisions made at the end of life. If all of the fetuses are equally viable, the abortions must be done on a random basis. To avoid the necessity of selective abortion as much as possible, the Conservative Movement's Committee on Jewish Law and Standards has ruled that only three zygotes should be implanted at one time.[47]

Surrogate Motherhood

This is really two different forms of overcoming infertility: "traditional surrogacy" or "ovum-surrogacy," in which the surrogate mother's own egg is fertilized by the sperm of the man in the couple who are trying to have a baby (presumably not the husband of the surrogate); and "gestational surrogacy," in which both the egg and the sperm are those of the couple, and the surrogate mother's womb is used to carry and deliver the baby.

This method of overcoming infertility, or at least something much akin to it, is among the oldest ways recorded in the Jewish tradition. Sarai (later, Sarah), after all, gives her handmaid, Hagar, to Abram (later, Abraham) specifically to conceive a son who would be attributed to Sarai, and Rachel and Leah likewise have their handmaids conceive children with their husband, Jacob. Leah, in fact, had already borne four sons by the time that she uses a surrogate mother because "she stopped bearing"—although she herself was later to bear him two more sons and a daughter.[48] These are all, in modern terminology, ovum-surrogates, and even so, because the handmaid belonged to the man's wife, the Bible attributes the child to the wife rather than the surrogate.

These precedents notwithstanding, though, surrogate motherhood raises difficult emotional and legal problems—although not technological problems beyond those of artificial insemination (in ovum-surrogacy) or in vitro fertilization (in gestational surrogacy). Thus rabbis raise some concerns about the way in which a surrogacy arrangement should be handled, but they do not ultimately prohibit it. Specifically, the couple must abide by civil law in their region and, in light of the newness of this matter in most systems of law, the couple must be informed of the possibility of legal challenges. Furthermore, Jewish law would require that steps be taken to insure that the surrogate mother has full and informed intent to abide by the agreement—perhaps, in ovum-surrogacy, at least, by giving her a period of time (usually thirty days) after birth to cancel the agreement. The surrogate mother must not have physical or other conditions that would make pregnancy dangerous for her beyond the risks normally associated with pregnancy. In ovum-surrogacy, the child must either be told the identity of the woman whose gametes he or she inherited or at least be given enough information to be able to avoid incest in his or her own sexual relations and to know about his or her physical and characterological background. Within these parameters, the few rabbis who have written about this have generally permitted surrogacy.[49]

Prenatal Diagnosis and Treatment; Gender Selection

Both for their own good and for that of their fetuses, pregnant women should seek and get prenatal care. They should also take the preventive measures that modern medicine prescribes to insure a healthy baby. These include restrictions on alcohol, smoking, and some prescription drugs; avoidance of toxins (e.g., in paints) and people with diseases that have been shown to cause fetal damage (e.g., German measles); and adoption of generally health-promoting habits of eating, hygiene, exercise, and sleep.

If the age or genetic background of a couple puts the child at risk for a degenerative, fatal genetic disease (e.g., Tay-Sachs) or for being seriously malformed, the mother may—but not must—undergo prenatal testing even though that puts the fetus at some risk. Moreover, if the tests reveal that the fetus suffers from such maladies, the mother may choose to abort it. If, however, techniques exist that can cure the child in utero or once born, she may, and probably should, choose to employ those techniques rather than abort the fetus.

According to all interpreters of Jewish law, it is generally not permissible to screen specifically for gender just because one wants a boy or a girl or to screen for any characteristic other than disease (e.g., height, intelligence). Similarly, the new sperm-splitting machine (a flow cytometer) to enable couples to choose either a boy or girl would generally violate Judaism's appreciation of people of both genders as equally created by God in the divine image.[50] At the same time, Jewish law, as noted earlier, requires a man to father at least two children, specifically a boy and a girl. While that could not be used to justify aborting a fetus of the same gender as the those already born, it might justify using the flow cytometer in families who have produced three or more children of one gender and none of the other.

Gene Therapy, Genetic Engineering, and Cloning

Gene therapy and genetic engineering are very new and only available in limited medical contexts. So, for example, techniques of genetic engineering are already being used to cure hydrocephalus while the fetus is still within the womb of the mother. There is already general agreement among rabbis that the legitimacy of human intervention to effect cure extends to procedures within the womb as well.[51] When used in this therapeutic way, genetic engineering is an unmitigated blessing.

The same techniques may potentially be used, however, to screen out traits that are not manifestations of a disease at all but merely characteristics that are deemed undesirable by certain individuals or groups. Abortion to eliminate defective fetuses poses the danger of the slippery slope where the definition of "defective" is broadened to the point of allowing only "perfect" children to be born, thus creating a master race. Genetic engineering gives us even more sophisticated tools to do this, for once we have the capability of changing not only the genes of a particular fetus but even its germ line, we are in a position to alter human descendance for all generations. That, of course, holds out the promise of rooting out genetic tendencies to heart disease, alcoholism, and a host of other medical problems, but it also will enable us to change the genetic traits of shortness, merely average intelligence, a particular skin color, and, perhaps, homosexuality. Moreover, genetic engineering will create a new organism, and that poses real risks to human beings and to the environment.

There are thus some uses of genetic engineering that are clearly legitimate or illegitimate, but there are many where it is, and will be, difficult to tell. How do we determine when we are using genetic engineering appropriately to aid God in ongoing, divine acts of cure and creation, and when, on the other hand, we are usurping the proper prerogatives of God to determine the nature of creation? More bluntly, when do we cease to act as the servants of God and pretend instead to be God?

Although cloning has been much more thoroughly discussed in the media, it actually presents fewer moral problems for Jews than genetic engineering does. Cloning, after all, does not introduce into the environment any new organism; it just replicates an organism that already exists, thus posing lesser risks. If cloning is used to overcome infertility, to aid in the research of diseases, or, in plants and animals, to produce food for starving people, it will be a very positive thing. On the other hand, cloning to avoid the intimacy of sexual intercourse, to gain immortality (as if that were possible through this technique), or to replicate oneself without any admixture of someone else's genes would be illegitimate uses of the technique. They smack of self-idolization and of the denial of human mortality; they thus make the moral and theological error of pretending that human beings are God.

Our moral doubts about genetic engineering and cloning do not mean that research into these techniques should stop; the potential benefits to our life and health are enormous. They should prompt us, however, to exercise care in how we use our new capabilities. The problems are not just medical and technological; they are moral and theological, requiring us to reexamine the very ways we understand ourselves as human beings, our relationships to each other and to God, and the limits inherent in being human.

Stem Cell Research

Jewish Views of Genetic Materials

Since human embryonic stem cells can be procured from aborted fetuses, the status of abortion within Judaism immediately arises. As we have seen, sometimes abortion is required by Jewish law and sometimes it is permitted, but mostly it is forbidden. The upshot of the Jewish stance on abortion, then, is that *if* a fetus was aborted for legitimate reasons under Jewish law, the aborted fetus may be used to advance our efforts to preserve the life and health of others.

In general, when a person dies, we must show honor to God's body by burying it as soon after death as possible. To benefit the lives of others, though, autopsies may be performed when the cause of death is not fully understood, and organ transplants are allowed to enable other people to live.[52] The fetus, though, does not have the status of a full-fledged human being. Therefore, if we can use the bodies of human beings to enable others to live, how much the more so may we use a part of a body—in this case, the "water" or "thigh" that constitutes the fetus—for that purpose. This all presumes, though, that the fetus was aborted for good and sufficient reason within the parameters of Jewish law.

Stem cells for research purposes can also be procured from donated sperm and eggs mixed together in a petri dish and cultured there. Genetic materials outside the uterus have no legal status in Jewish law, for they are not even a part of a human being until implanted in a woman's womb and even then, during the first forty days of gestation, their status is "as if they were simply water."[53] Abortion is still prohibited during that time except for therapeutic purposes, for in the uterus such gametes have the potential of growing into a human being, but outside the womb, at least as of now, they have no such potential. As a result, frozen embryos may be discarded or used for reasonable purposes, and so may stem cells procured from them.

Other Factors in Stem Cell Research

Given that the materials for stem cell research can be procured in permissible ways, the technology itself is morally neutral. It gains its moral valence on the basis of what we do with it. The question, then, reduces to a risk-benefit analysis of stem cell research. The articles in a recent *Hastings Center Report*[54] raise some questions to be considered in such an analysis, and I will not rehearse them here. I want to note only two things about them from a Jewish perspective:

First, the Jewish tradition sees the provision of health care as a communal responsibility, and so the justice arguments in the *Hastings Center Report* have a special resonance for me as a Jew. Especially since much of the basic science in this area was funded by the government, the government has the right to require private companies to provide their applications of that science to those who cannot afford them at reduced rates or, if necessary, even for free. At the same time, the Jewish tradition does not demand socialism, and for many good reasons, we, in the United States, have adopted a modified, capitalistic system of economics. The trick, then, will be to balance access to applications of the new technology with the legitimate right of a private company to make a profit on its efforts to develop and market applications of stem cell research.

Second, the potential of stem cell research for creating organs for transplant and cures for diseases is, at least in theory, both awesome and hopeful. Indeed, in light of our divine mandate to seek to maintain life and health, one might even argue that from a Jewish perspective we have a *duty* to proceed with that research. As difficult as it may be, though, we must draw a clear line between uses of this or any other technology for cure, which are to be applauded, as against uses of this technology for enhancement, which must be approached with extreme caution. Jews have been the brunt of campaigns of positive eugenics both here, in the United States, and in Nazi Germany,[55] and so we are especially sensitive to creating a model human being that is to be replicated through the genetic engineering that stem cell applications will involve. Moreover, when Jews see a disabled human being, we are not to recoil from the disability or count our blessings for not being disabled in that way; we are rather commanded to recite a blessing thanking God for making people different.[56] In light, then, of the Jewish view that all human beings are created in the image of God, regardless of their levels of ability or disability, it is imperative from a Jewish perspective that the applications of stem cell research be used for cure and not for enhancement.

My recommendation, then, is that we take the steps necessary to advance stem cell research and its applications in an effort to take advantage of its great potential for good. We should do so, though, with restrictions to enable access to its applications to all Americans who need it and to prohibit applications intended to make all human beings into any particular model of human excellence. Instead, through this technology and all others, we should seek to cure diseases while simultaneously retaining our appreciation for the variety of God's creatures.

NOTES

1. This essay is excerpted and slightly revised from a longer entry, "Religious Views on Biotechnology: Jewish," in the *Encyclopedia of Ethical, Legal, and Policy Issues in Biotechnology*, ed. Thomas H. Murray and Maxwell Mehleman, pp. 924–38, copyright © 2000 by John Wiley & Sons, Inc. Reprinted by permission of John Wiley & Sons, Inc.

2. Those interested in at least one Jewish approach to issues at the end of life and to a more expanded treatment of issues at the beginning of life may consult my book, *Matters of Life and Death: A Jewish Approach to Modern Medical Ethics* (Philadelphia: Jewish Publication Society, 1998).

3. See, for example, Deuteronomy 10:14; Psalms 24:1. See also Genesis 14:19, 22 (where the Hebrew word for "Creator" [*koneh*] also means "Possessor," and where "heaven and earth" is a merism for those and everything in between); Exodus 20:11; Leviticus 25:23, 42, 55; Deuteronomy 4:35, 39; 32:6.

4. *Genesis Rabbah* 11:6; *Pesikta Rabbati* 22:4.

5. In my book on Jewish medical ethics, I identify and discuss seven such underlying principles, but the three I name here will suffice for our purposes in this chapter. For further discussion on these three and for a description of the four others, see Dorff, *Matters of Life and Death*, ch. 2.

6. Thus, for example, bathing is a commandment, according to Hillel: *Leviticus Rabbah* 34:3. Maimonides includes rules requiring proper care of the body in his code of Jewish law as a positive obligation (not just advice for feeling good or living a long life), parallel to the positive duty to aid the poor: M.T. *Laws of Ethics (De'ot)*, chs. 3–5.

7. B. *Shabbat* 32a; B. *Bava Kamma* 15b, 80a, 91b; M.T. *Laws of Murder* 11:4–5; S.A. *Yoreh De'ah* 116:5 gloss; S.A. *Hoshen Mishpat* 427:8–10. Jewish law views endangering one's health as worse than violating a ritual prohibition: B. *Hullin* 10a; S.A. *Orah Hayyim* 173:2; S.A. *Yoreh De'ah* 116:5 gloss.

8. For the opinions of Rabbi J. David Bleich (Orthodox), Rabbi Solomon Freehof (Reform), and the Rabbi Seymour Siegel (Conservative), as well as a resolution of the (Conservative) Rabbinical Assembly, see Elliot N. Dorff and Arthur Rosett, *A Living Tree: The Roots and Growth of Jewish Law* (Albany: State University of New York Press, 1988), pp. 337–62.

9. Genesis 9:5; M. *Semahot* 2:2; B. *Bava Kamma* 91b; *Genesis Rabbah* 34:19 states that the ban against suicide includes not only cases where blood was shed, but also self-inflicted death through strangulation and the like; M.T. *Laws of Murder* 2:3; M.T. *Laws of Injury and Damage* 5:1; S.A. *Yoreh De'ah* 345:1–3. Cf. J. David Bleich, *Judaism and Healing* (New York: Ktav, 1981), ch. 26.

10. The Rabbis note that the Nazarite, who takes an oath to avoid such pleasures, must, according to Numbers 6:11, bring a sin offering after the time specified by his oath, and they derive from that law that abstinence is prohibited: B. *Ta'anit* 11a. Cf. also M.T. *Laws of Ethics (De'ot)* 3:1.

11. M.T. *Laws of Ethics (De'ot)* 3:3.

12. *Sifra* on Leviticus 19:16; B. *Sanhedrin* 73a; M.T. *Laws of Murder* 1:14; S.A. *Hoshen Mishpat* 426.

13. E.g., Exodus 15:26; Deuteronomy 32:39; Isaiah 19:22; 57:18–19; Jeremiah 30:17; 33:6; Hosea 6:1; Psalms 103:2–3; 107:20; Job 5:18.

14. The permission and duty to heal: B. *Bava Kamma* 85a, 81b; B. *Sanhedrin* 73a, 84b (with Rashi's commentary there). See also *Sifrei Deuteronomy* on Deuteronomy 22:2 and *Leviticus Rabbah* 34:3. Nahmanides, *Kitvei Haramban*, Bernard Chavel, ed. (Jerusalem: Mosad Harav Kook, 1963 [Hebrew]), Vol. 2, p. 43, bases the duty for the community to provide health care on Leviticus 19:18, "You shall love your neighbor as yourself"; this passage comes from Nahmanides' *Torat Ha'adam (The Instruction of Man)*, Sh'ar Sakkanah (Section on Danger) on B. *Bava Kamma*, ch. 8, and is cited by Joseph Karo in his commentary to the *Tur, Bet Yosef, Yoreh De'ah* 336. Nahmanides bases himself on similar reasoning in B. *Sanhedrin* 84b.

15. B. *Sanhedrin* 74a.

16. The best of physicians deserves to go to Hell: B. *Kiddushin* 82a. Abraham ibn Ezra, Bahya ibn Pakuda, and Jonathan Eybeschuetz all restricted the physician's mandate to external injuries: see Ibn Ezra's commentary on Exodus 21:19 and cf. his comments on Exodus 15:26 and 23:25, where he cites Job 5:18 and II Chronicles 16:12 in support of his view; Bahya's commentary on Exodus 21:19; and Eybeschuetz, *Kereti U'pleti* on S.A. *Yoreh De'ah* 188:5. See Immanuel Jakobovits, *Jewish Medical Ethics* (New York: Bloch, 1959, 1975), pp. 5–6. That a Jew may not live in a city without a physician: J. *Kiddushin* 66d; see also B. *Sanhedrin* 17b, where this requirement is applied only to "the students of the Sages."

17. S.A. *Yoreh De'ah* 336:1.

18. *Midrash Temurrah* as cited in *Otzar Midrashim*, J.D. Eisenstein, ed. (New York, 1915) II, 580–581. Cf. also B. *Avodah Zarah* 40b, a story in which Rabbi expresses appreciation for foods that can cure. Although circumcision is not justified in the Jewish tradition in medical terms, it is instructive that the rabbis maintained, as noted above, that Jewish boys were not born circumcised specifically because God created the world such that it would need human fixing, a similar idea to the one articulated here on behalf of physicians' activity despite God's rule; see note 2 above.

19. B. *Shabbat* 10a, 119b. In the first of those passages, it is the judge who judges justly who is called God's partner; in the second, it is anyone who recites Genesis 2:1–3 (about God resting on the seventh day) on Friday night who thereby participates in God's ongoing act of creation. The Talmud in B. *Sanhedrin* 38a specifically wanted the Sadducees *not* to be able to say that angels or any beings other than humans participate with God in creation.

20. On this entire matter, the Rabbinical Assembly, the rabbinic body of the Conservative Movement within Judaism, has created a rabbinic letter designed for use with adults and with teenagers discussing the concepts, values, and laws of Judaism governing intimate relations, marriage, non-marital sex, and homosexuality. See Elliot N. Dorff, *"This Is My Beloved, This Is My Friend": A Rabbinic Letter on Intimate Relations* (New York: Rabbinical Assembly, 1996). See also chs. 3–6 of my book, *Matters of Life and Death.*

21. Genesis 2:18; cf. *Midrash Psalms* on Psalms 59:2. Exodus 21:10 prescribes that a woman has conjugal rights in marriage, just as a man does, and the rabbis then spell out exactly how often a man must offer to have sex with his wife and how long she can refuse his advances without losing part of her settlement in a divorce; see note 4 above. Note that he may never force himself upon her.

22. For example, Deuteronomy 7:13–14; 28:4, 11; Psalms 128:6.

23. Genesis 15:5; 17:3–6, 15–21; 18:18; 28:14; 32:13.

24. M. *Yevamot* 6:6 (61b); B. *Yevamot* 65b–66a; M.T. *Laws of Marriage* 15:2; S.A. *Even Ha'ezer* 1:1, 13. That one should have as many children as possible: B. *Yevamost* 62b (based on the rabbis' interpretation of Isaiah 45:18 and Ecclesiastes 11:6); M.T. *Laws of Marriage* 15:16.

25. Deuteronomy 6:5.

26. B. *Yevamot* 12b. For a thorough discussion of this, see David M. Feldman, *Birth Control in Jewish Law* (New York: New York University Press, 1968); reprinted as *Marital Relations, Abortion, and Birth Control in Jewish Law* (New York: Schocken, 1973).

27. M.T. *Laws of Forbidden Intercourse* 16:2, 6; S.A. *Even Ha'ever* 5:2.

28. B. *Shabbat* 110b.

29. Bleich, *Judaism and Healing*, p. 65; David Feldman and Fred Rosner, eds., *Compendium on Medical Ethics* (New York: Federation of Jewish Philanthropies, 1984), pp. 46–47; Solomon Freehof, *Reform Responsa* (Cincinnati, Ohio: Hebrew Union College Press, 1960), pp. 206–8.

30. B. *Yevamot* 69b. Rabbi Immanuel Jakobovits, *Jewish Medical Ethics*, p. 275, notes that "forty days" in talmudic terms may mean just under two months in our modern way of calculating gestation. See note 53 below. First trimester: B. *Niddah* 17a.

31. B. *Hullin* 58a and elsewhere.

32. Feldman, *Birth Control in Jewish Law*, pp. 265–66 and ch. 15.

33. M. *Niddah* 3:5.

34. M. *Oholot* 7:6. There are variant versions of this. Like our Mishnah, J. *Shabbat* 14:4 reads "its greater part"; T. *Yevamot* 9:9 and B. *Sanhedrin* 72b have "its head;" and J. *Sanhedrin* 8, end, has "its head or its greater part."

35. Jakobovits, *Jewish Medical Ethics,* pp. 186–187 and pp. 378–79, n. 173.

36. Feldman, *Birth Control in Jewish Law*, pp. 284–94; Moshe Halevi Spero, *Judaism and Psychology: Halakhic Perspectives* (New York: Ktav, 1980), ch. 12.

37. Feldman, *Birth Control in Jewish Law*, pp. 284–94, and Jakobovits, *Jewish Medical Ethics*, pp. 189–190.

38. J. David Bleich, *Contemporary Halakhic Problems* (New York: Ktav, 1977), pp. 112–15; J. David Bleich, in Rosner and Bleich, eds., *Jewish Bioethics* (New York: Sanhedrin Press, 1979), Ch. 9, esp. pp. 161 and 175, n. 97.

39. Feldman, *Birth Control in Jewish Law*, pp. 284–94.

40. Eliezer Waldenberg, *Responsa Tzitz Eliezer*, 9:51 (1967) and 13:102 (1978) [Hebrew]; S. Israeli, *Amud Hayemini*, no. 35 cited in *No'am*, vol. 16 (K.H.), p. 27 (note) [Hebrew]; Lev Grossnass, *Responsa Lev Aryeh* 2:205 [Hebrew]; Alex J. Goldman, *Judaism Confronts Contemporary Issues* (New York: Ktav, 1978), Ch. 3, esp. pp. 52–62.

41. Jakobovits, *Jewish Medical Ethics*, p. 264; Bleich, *Judaism and Healing*, pp. 82–84.

42. Bleich, *Judaism and Healing*, pp. 80–84, cites five prominent Orthodox authorities as requiring physical contact of the genital organs for adultery to occur. Nevertheless, as he points out, these Orthodox rabbis would prohibit donor insemination on the grounds of potential incest in the next generation, as discussed in the next paragraph. Moreover, some Orthodox rabbis Bleich cites maintain that violating the prohibition against adultery does not require genital contact, and so they would object to donor insemination on that ground as well.

43. Elliot N. Dorff, "Artificial Insemination, Egg Donation, and Adoption," *Conservative Judaism* 49, no. 1 (1996): pp. 3–60. This rabbinic ruling, approved in 1994 by the Conservative Movement's Committee on Jewish Law and Standards, also discusses several ancillary concerns, such as the identity of the father for various purposes in Jewish law; the psychological issues raised by the asymmetry in the situation—namely, that the child will be the biological product of the woman but not the man who will be raising him/her; and the psychological need of the child to know his/her genetic roots. This ruling was reprinted in Dorff, *Matters of Life and Death*, pp. 66–115.

44. Robert Spirtas, Steven C. Kaufman, and Nancy J. Alexander, *Fertility and Sterility* [the journal of the American Fertility Society] 59, no. 2 (1993): 291–92. I want to thank my friend, Dr. Michael Grodin, for sharing this article with me. The 1988 Congressional report also reported a number of other possible complications caused by commonly used drugs to stimulate the ovaries, including early pregnancy loss, multiple gestations (fetuses), ectopic pregnancies, headache, hair loss, pleuropulmonary fibrosis, increased blood viscosity and hypertension, stroke, and myocardial infarction; see U.S. Congress, Office of Technology Assessment, *Infertility: Medical and Social Choices*, OTA-BA-358 (Washington, D.C.: U.S. Government Printing Office, May 1988), pp. 128–129. Once again, though, the demonstrated risks are not so great as to make stimulation of the ovaries for egg donation prohibited as a violation of the Jewish command to guard our health, but they are sufficient to demand that caution be taken and that the number of times a woman donates eggs be limited.

45. Rabbi Aaron Mackler, "In Vitro Fertilization," in *Life and Death Responsibilities in Jewish Biomedical Ethics*, ed. Aaron L. Mackler (New York: Jewish Theological Seminary of America, 2000), pp. 97–122, esp. pp. 108–110 and 113.

46. See, for example, Bleich, *Judaism and Healing*, pp. 85–91; and Dorff, "Artificial Insemination," pp. 17–18, 47–48 (with regard to donor insemination and egg donation, but the same considerations, although sometimes in different forms, apply to IVF, GIFT, and ZIFT). See also Dorff, *Matters of Life and Death*, chs. 3 and 4.

47. Dorff, "Artificial Insemination," p. 47. Dorff, *Matters of Life and Death*, pp. 56–57, 101–102, 129–30.

48. Genesis 16:2 uses a play on words in Hebrew when Sarai says to Abram, "Look, the Lord has kept me from bearing. Consort with my maid [Hagar]; perhaps I shall have a son [also, I shall be built up] through her." This indicates that Ishmael, the son that resulted from this union, was not only to be considered Abram's son, but Sarai's as well. Similarly, Rachel tells Jacob,

"Here is my maid Bilhah. Consort with her, that she may bear on my knees and that through her I too may have children" (Genesis 30:3). At that time, Rachel was infertile (she gave birth to Joseph and Benjamin only later), but Leah, who had already had four sons, also gave her handmaid, Zilpah, to Jacob, and when Zilpah bore two sons to Jacob, Leah says " 'What fortune!' meaning, 'Women will deem me fortunate' " (Genesis 30:13)—indicating that those two sons were ascribed to Leah as well. That Leah had stopped bearing and therefore resorts to the use of her handmaid Zilpah: Genesis 30:9. That she later bears three more children: Genesis 30:14–21.

49. See, for example, Bleich, *Judaism and Healing*, pp. 92–95. While Rabbi Bleich generally prohibits or limits the use of new medical procedures, here he specifically argues against Rabbi Jakobovits' claim that surrogacy is inherently immoral and spends most of his discussion on the question of the Jewish identity of the child. See also Michael Gold, *And Hannah Wept: Infertility, Adoption, and the Jewish Couple* (Philadelphia: Jewish Publication Society, 1988), pp. 120–27; and Elie Spitz, "On the Birth of Surrogates," in *Life and Death Responsibilities in Jewish Biomedical Ethics*, ed. Aaron L. Mackler (New York: Jewish Theological Seminary of America, 2000), pp. 129–61. Rabbi Spitz's rabbinic ruling was approved by the Conservative Movement's Committee on Jewish Law and Standards in September 1997.

50. For a good, popular article describing some of the issues involved, see Lisa Belkin, "Getting the Girl," *New York Times Magazine*, 25 July 1999, pp. 26–31, 38, 54–55.

51. For example, Bleich, *Judaism and Healing*, p. 106.

52. For classical sources on this, see Dorff, *Matters of Life and Death*, ch. 9.

53. B. *Yevamot* 69b. Rabbi Immanuel Jakobovits notes that "forty days" in talmudic terms may mean just under two months in our modern way of calculating gestation since the Rabbis counted from the time of the first missed menstrual flow while we count from the time of conception, approximately two weeks earlier. See Jakobovits, *Jewish Medical Ethics*, p. 275.

54. See *Hastings Center Report* 29, no. 2 (1999): 30–48.

55. See Stephen J. Gould, *The Mismeasure of Man* (New York: W. W. Norton and Company, Inc., 1996), and George J. Annas and Michael A. Grodin, *The Nazi Doctors and the Nuremberg Code: Human Rights in Human Experimentation* (New York: Oxford University Press, 1992).

56. For a thorough discussion of this blessing and concept in Jewish tradition, see Carl Astor, ". . . *Who Makes People Different": Jewish Perspectives on the Disabled* (New York: United Synagogue of America, 1985).

Contributors

Courtney Campbell is an associate professor of philosophy at Oregon State University in Corvallis, Oregon.

Audrey R. Chapman is program director of the Program of Dialogue on Science, Ethics, and Religion, and the Science and Human Rights Program of the Directorate for Science and Policy Programs of the American Association for the Advancement of Science in Washington, D.C.

Ronald Cole-Turner is the H. Parker Sharp Professor of Theology and Ethics at Pittsburgh Theological Seminary in Pittsburgh, Pennsylvania.

Elliot N. Dorff is rector and Distinguished Professor of Philosophy at the University of Judaism in Los Angeles, California, and is vice chair of the Conservative Movement's Committee on Jewish Law and Standards.

John H. Evans is an assistant professor of sociology at the University of California, San Diego.

Mark J. Hanson is the executive director of the Missoula Demonstration Project, a research faculty member in the Department of Philosophy at the University of Montana in Missoula, and a faculty associate at its Practical Ethics Center. He is the former associate for Ethics and Society at The Hastings Center in Garrison, New York.

B. Andrew Lustig is director of the Program on Biotechnology, Religion, and Ethics, and a research scholar in the religious studies department at Rice University in Houston, Texas.

Gerald P. McKenny is an associate professor of theological ethics at the University of Notre Dame in Notre Dame, Indiana.

Index